The Complete Guide to Dermatopathology for Students

CARROL

The Complete Guide to Dermatopathology for Students

Copyright © 2023 by CARROL

The first edition was published in 2023

ISBN:
Published by:
Sunshine
1663 Liberty Drive
Hyderabad, IN 47403
www.Sunshinepublishers.com

This book is self-published using on-demand printing and publishing, which allows it to be printed and distributed globally

TABLE OF CONTENT

Chapter 4: Dermatopathological Examination 28

Chapter 5: Inflammatory Skin Disorders 36

Chapter 6: Infectious Skin Conditions 46

Chapter 7: Neoplastic Skin Conditions   54

Chapter 8: Autoimmune and Connective Tissue Disorders   64

Chapter 9: Special Techniques in Dermatopathology   72

Chapter 10: Dermatopathology in Clinical Practice 78

Dermatopathology in Dermatology Clinics

Dermatopathology in Surgical Pathology

Dermatopathology in Research

Chapter 11: Case Studies in Dermatopathology 85

Case Study 1: Inflammatory Skin Disorder

Case Study 2: Infectious Skin Condition

Case Study 3: Neoplastic Skin Condition

Case Study 4: Autoimmune and Connective Tissue Disorder

Chapter 12: Future Directions in Dermatopathology 93

Advances in Dermatopathological Techniques

Emerging Trends in Dermatopathology Research

Role of Artificial Intelligence in Dermatopathology

Chapter 1: Introduction to Dermatopathology

Understanding Dermatopathology

Dermatopathology is a specialized field within dermatology that focuses on the study and diagnosis of skin diseases through the examination of skin tissue samples. It is a crucial aspect of dermatology as it provides valuable insights into the underlying causes and mechanisms of various skin conditions. In this subchapter, we aim to provide students with a comprehensive understanding of dermatopathology and its significance in the field of dermatology.

To begin with, dermatopathology involves the analysis of skin biopsies, which are small pieces of skin tissue removed for examination under a microscope. These biopsies are obtained through various techniques, such as punch biopsies, excisional biopsies, or shave biopsies. Once the samples are collected, they are processed, stained, and examined by dermatopathologists, who are specially trained physicians with expertise in both dermatology and pathology.

The primary goal of dermatopathology is to establish an accurate diagnosis by analyzing the structural and cellular changes within the skin tissue. This involves identifying the presence of abnormal cells, inflammation, infections, tumors, and other pathological changes. Through detailed examination, dermatopathologists can determine the nature of the disease, its severity, and potential treatment options.

In addition to diagnosis, dermatopathology also plays a vital role in monitoring disease progression and response to treatment. By comparing biopsies taken at different time points, dermatologists can assess the effectiveness of therapeutic interventions and make adjustments as necessary. This aspect of dermatopathology is particularly important in chronic skin diseases, such as psoriasis or eczema, where long-term management is required.

Moreover, dermatopathology contributes to the advancement of medical knowledge and research. By studying skin biopsies, researchers can uncover new insights into the pathogenesis of various skin diseases, identify novel therapeutic targets, and develop more effective treatment strategies. This research is crucial for improving patient care and expanding the understanding of dermatological conditions.

In conclusion, dermatopathology is a fundamental discipline within dermatology that enables the accurate diagnosis, monitoring, and research of skin diseases. By understanding the principles and techniques of dermatopathology, students can enhance their diagnostic skills and contribute to the field of dermatology. With its interdisciplinary nature, dermatopathology offers a bridge between clinical dermatology and anatomical pathology, providing a comprehensive approach to the study and management of skin disorders.

Importance of Dermatopathology for Students

The field of dermatopathology plays a vital role in the study and practice of dermatology. As students pursuing a career in dermatology, it is crucial to understand the importance of dermatopathology and how it contributes to our understanding and diagnosis of various skin conditions. In this subchapter, we will delve into the significance of dermatopathology for students in the field of dermatology.

Dermatopathology, at its core, is the study of skin diseases through the examination of skin tissue samples. It combines the knowledge of both dermatology and pathology, providing a comprehensive understanding of skin disorders. By studying dermatopathology, students can develop a deeper understanding of the underlying histopathological changes that occur in different skin diseases.

One of the primary benefits of dermatopathology for students lies in its ability to enhance diagnostic skills. By examining tissue samples under a microscope, students can identify specific patterns and characteristics associated with different skin disorders. This knowledge is crucial in accurately diagnosing and treating patients. Dermatopathology allows students to bridge the gap between clinical presentation and histological findings, ensuring accurate diagnoses and appropriate management plans.

Additionally, studying dermatopathology enables students to gain a solid foundation in basic pathological concepts. Understanding the cellular and molecular changes in skin diseases is essential in providing effective treatment options and predicting disease progression. Dermatopathology equips students with the knowledge to interpret laboratory reports and collaborate effectively with pathologists in interdisciplinary settings.

Moreover, dermatopathology fosters critical thinking skills among students. It encourages them to analyze and interpret complex histological findings, integrating clinical information to arrive at accurate diagnoses. This analytical approach is essential in the field of dermatology, where conditions can often present with similar clinical features.

Lastly, dermatopathology allows students to contribute to the advancement of dermatology through research and academic pursuits. By staying updated on the latest developments in dermatopathology, students can actively participate in scientific discussions, publish papers, and present their findings at conferences.

In conclusion, dermatopathology is of utmost importance for students in the field of dermatology. It enhances diagnostic skills, provides a solid foundation in pathology, fosters critical thinking, and allows students to contribute to the field's advancement. Embracing dermatopathology as an integral part of our education will undoubtedly help us become competent and knowledgeable future dermatologists.

Scope of Dermatopathology in Medical Education

Dermatopathology is a specialized field within dermatology that combines the study of both dermatology and pathology. It focuses on the diagnosis and understanding of skin diseases through the examination of skin tissue samples under a microscope. In today's rapidly evolving medical landscape, the scope of dermatopathology has expanded, making it an essential component of medical education for students interested in dermatology.

The field of dermatopathology offers students a unique opportunity to gain a comprehensive understanding of various skin diseases. By analyzing skin tissue samples, students can learn to identify the microscopic features of different skin conditions, such as inflammatory disorders, infectious diseases, and neoplastic processes. This knowledge allows for accurate diagnosis and appropriate treatment planning, ultimately leading to better patient outcomes.

Incorporating dermatopathology into medical education provides students with a holistic approach to dermatology. It enhances their ability to correlate clinical findings with histopathological changes, enabling a deeper understanding of the underlying mechanisms of skin diseases. By integrating dermatopathology into their education, students will develop the skills necessary to effectively communicate with pathologists and collaborate in interdisciplinary teams.

Furthermore, the scope of dermatopathology extends beyond traditional histopathological examination. Technological advancements have brought about innovative techniques such as immunohistochemistry, molecular diagnostics, and genetic testing.

These tools enable students to delve deeper into the molecular and genetic basis of skin diseases, leading to more accurate diagnoses and personalized treatment plans.

In addition to diagnostic skills, dermatopathology also equips students with research opportunities. By analyzing skin tissue samples, students can contribute to the advancement of scientific knowledge in dermatology. Through research projects, students can explore new diagnostic and therapeutic modalities, contributing to the development of novel treatment strategies.

To fully grasp the scope of dermatopathology, medical education should incorporate both didactic and hands-on experiences. Didactic lectures and interactive sessions can provide students with a solid foundation in the principles and theories of dermatopathology. Practical training, such as microscopy sessions and supervised analysis of histopathological slides, allows students to develop the necessary technical skills and interpretative abilities.

In conclusion, dermatopathology plays a crucial role in medical education for students interested in dermatology. It offers a comprehensive understanding of skin diseases, enhances diagnostic skills, facilitates interdisciplinary collaboration, and provides research opportunities. By incorporating dermatopathology into medical curricula, students will be well-prepared to tackle the challenges of diagnosing and managing various skin conditions, ultimately improving patient care in the field of dermatology.

Chapter 2: Basics of Dermatopathology

Skin Anatomy and Physiology

As students of dermatology, it is crucial to have a thorough understanding of the skin's anatomy and physiology. The skin is the largest organ of the body and plays a vital role in protecting us from external factors, regulating body temperature, and providing sensory information. This subchapter aims to provide you with a comprehensive overview of the skin's structure and its physiological functions.

The skin consists of three main layers: the epidermis, dermis, and subcutaneous tissue. The epidermis, the outermost layer, is composed of several layers of cells, primarily keratinocytes. These cells constantly undergo a process called keratinization, where they harden and form a protective barrier against environmental factors. The epidermis also contains melanocytes, responsible for producing melanin, the pigment that gives color to our skin.

Beneath the epidermis lies the dermis, which is a much thicker layer. It is composed of connective tissue, blood vessels, nerve endings, and various appendages such as hair follicles and sweat glands. The dermis provides structural support to the skin and houses important components like collagen and elastin, which give the skin its strength and elasticity.

The subcutaneous tissue, also known as the hypodermis, lies below the dermis and is primarily composed of fat cells. It acts as an insulator, helping to regulate body temperature and providing cushioning and protection to deeper structures.

Understanding the physiology of the skin is equally important. The skin has multiple functions, including protection, sensation, thermoregulation, and excretion. It acts as a physical barrier, preventing the entry of harmful microorganisms and chemicals into the body. The skin also contains sensory receptors that allow us to perceive touch, pressure, temperature, and pain.

One of the skin's key roles is thermoregulation, as it helps maintain body temperature within a narrow range. When the body is too hot, sweat glands produce sweat that evaporates, cooling the skin. In colder conditions, blood vessels constrict to reduce heat loss, and the contraction of muscles generates heat.

Additionally, the skin plays a role in excretion, as small amounts of waste products and toxins are eliminated through sweat glands.

In conclusion, understanding the anatomy and physiology of the skin is essential for students of dermatology. The skin's complex structure and functions form the basis for diagnosing and treating various skin conditions. By delving into the intricacies of skin anatomy and physiology, students will develop a solid foundation to further explore the fascinating field of dermatopathology.

Common Skin Disorders

In the field of dermatology, it is essential for students to have a comprehensive understanding of the various skin disorders that they may encounter in their practice. This subchapter aims to provide students with an overview of some of the most common skin disorders, their causes, symptoms, and treatment options.

1. Acne: Acne is a chronic inflammatory skin condition that affects millions of people worldwide. It is characterized by the presence of pimples, blackheads, and whiteheads. The primary cause of acne is the overproduction of oil by the sebaceous glands, which leads to clogged pores. Treatment options include topical or oral medications, lifestyle modifications, and cosmetic procedures.

2. Eczema: Eczema, also known as atopic dermatitis, is a chronic condition that causes dry, itchy, and inflamed skin. It often appears in childhood and can persist into adulthood. The exact cause of eczema is unknown, but it is believed to involve a combination of genetic and environmental factors. Treatment includes moisturizers, topical corticosteroids, and avoiding triggers.

3. Psoriasis: Psoriasis is a chronic autoimmune disease characterized by red, scaly patches on the skin. It is caused by an overactive immune system that speeds up the skin cell turnover process. Treatment options include topical medications, phototherapy, and systemic medications.

4. Rosacea: Rosacea is a common chronic skin condition that primarily affects the face. It is characterized by redness, small blood vessels, and often, acne-like bumps. The exact cause of rosacea is unknown, but

triggers such as sun exposure, spicy foods, and alcohol can exacerbate the condition. Treatment includes topical or oral medications, laser therapy, and lifestyle modifications.

5. Dermatitis: Dermatitis refers to inflammation of the skin and can be caused by various factors, including allergens, irritants, and genetic predisposition. The symptoms may include redness, itching, and rash. Treatment options include topical corticosteroids, antihistamines, and avoiding triggers.

6. Melanoma: Melanoma is a type of skin cancer that develops from pigment-producing cells called melanocytes. It is often caused by exposure to ultraviolet (UV) radiation from the sun or tanning beds. Early detection and treatment are crucial for a favorable prognosis. Treatment options may include surgery, radiation therapy, and targeted therapy.

By familiarizing themselves with these common skin disorders, students will be better equipped to identify, diagnose, and treat patients. It is important to note that while this subchapter provides an overview, the complete understanding of each disorder requires further study and clinical experience. Dermatology is a dynamic field, and ongoing research and advancements continue to shape the diagnosis and management of these skin disorders.

Histopathological Techniques in Dermatopathology

In the field of dermatopathology, histopathological techniques play a crucial role in the accurate diagnosis and treatment of various skin diseases. This subchapter aims to provide students with an in-depth understanding of the histopathological techniques commonly used in dermatology.

Histopathology is the microscopic examination of tissue samples to study the structural changes that occur in diseases. In dermatopathology, skin biopsies are obtained and processed using specific techniques to visualize the cellular and tissue changes associated with dermatological conditions.

One of the most commonly used techniques is the Hematoxylin and Eosin (H&E) staining. This staining method allows for the visualization of cellular structures and differentiates between various tissue components such as nuclei, cytoplasm, and connective tissue. H&E staining is critical in identifying characteristic features of skin diseases, including inflammatory infiltrates, abnormal cell growth, and pigmentary changes.

Immunohistochemistry (IHC) is another vital technique used in dermatopathology. By employing specific antibodies, IHC helps identify proteins and other cellular markers that are present in different skin diseases. This technique aids in differentiating between various types of skin cancers and inflammatory conditions, as well as determining the prognosis and guiding treatment decisions.

Special staining techniques, such as periodic acid-Schiff (PAS) and Giemsa staining, are also commonly employed in dermatopathology.

PAS staining is useful in identifying fungal infections, while Giemsa staining is effective in diagnosing conditions like leishmaniasis and certain types of skin tumors.

In addition to staining techniques, dermatopathologists also utilize various tissue processing methods. Frozen section technique allows for rapid examination of tissue samples during surgery, providing immediate feedback to the surgeon. This technique is particularly helpful in Mohs micrographic surgery, a specialized technique for removing skin cancers with minimal tissue loss.

Moreover, electron microscopy is an advanced technique used in specific cases to study ultrastructural changes in skin diseases. It provides high-resolution images of cellular organelles, allowing for a detailed analysis of complex dermatological conditions.

Understanding and mastering these histopathological techniques are essential for students pursuing a career in dermatology. By utilizing these techniques, dermatopathologists can accurately diagnose skin diseases, determine appropriate treatment strategies, and contribute to improved patient outcomes.

In conclusion, the subchapter on histopathological techniques in dermatopathology provides students with a comprehensive overview of the essential techniques used in the field. By familiarizing themselves with these techniques, students will develop the necessary skills to analyze and interpret histopathological findings, contributing to their success in the field of dermatology.

Chapter 3: Skin Biopsies and Specimen Handling

Indications for Skin Biopsy

In the field of dermatology, skin biopsy plays a crucial role in the diagnosis and management of various skin conditions. A skin biopsy involves the removal of a small sample of skin tissue for microscopic examination and analysis. This diagnostic procedure is especially useful when the dermatologist needs to confirm or rule out a suspected skin disease or condition. In this subchapter, we will explore the indications for skin biopsy and shed light on how this procedure aids in the diagnosis and treatment of dermatological issues.

One of the primary indications for a skin biopsy is the evaluation of a suspicious skin lesion. Skin lesions that exhibit concerning features such as asymmetry, irregular borders, color variation, or rapid growth may warrant further investigation through a biopsy. By examining the skin tissue under a microscope, dermatopathologists can accurately diagnose conditions like melanoma, basal cell carcinoma, squamous cell carcinoma, and other types of skin cancers.

Skin biopsies are also valuable in diagnosing inflammatory skin conditions. Conditions such as psoriasis, eczema, lichen planus, and lupus erythematosus often present with characteristic changes in the skin. A biopsy can help confirm these diagnoses by identifying specific histopathological patterns associated with each condition. This information is crucial for selecting appropriate treatment options and monitoring disease progression.

Furthermore, skin biopsies can aid in diagnosing infectious skin diseases. Fungal, bacterial, and viral infections can cause a wide range of skin manifestations, including rashes, blisters, or nodules. By examining the skin tissue, dermatopathologists can identify the causative agent and prescribe the most effective antimicrobial or antiviral treatment.

In some cases, skin biopsies are performed to evaluate systemic diseases that have cutaneous manifestations. Conditions like systemic lupus erythematosus, sarcoidosis, or vasculitis can affect multiple organs, including the skin. Biopsies can help confirm the presence of specific histological changes associated with these diseases and guide appropriate treatment choices.

In conclusion, skin biopsy is a valuable diagnostic tool in dermatology. By examining skin tissue under a microscope, dermatopathologists can accurately diagnose various skin conditions, including skin cancers, inflammatory diseases, infectious diseases, and systemic diseases with cutaneous manifestations. Understanding the indications for skin biopsy is essential for students studying dermatology as it enables them to provide accurate diagnoses and develop appropriate treatment plans for their patients.

Different Types of Skin Biopsies

In the field of dermatology, skin biopsies play a crucial role in diagnosing various skin conditions and diseases. A skin biopsy involves the removal of a small sample of skin tissue for further examination under a microscope. This subchapter will provide an overview of the different types of skin biopsies commonly performed in dermatopathology, helping students gain a comprehensive understanding of this essential diagnostic procedure.

1. Punch Biopsy: This is the most commonly performed skin biopsy technique. It involves using a cylindrical tool to remove a small, circular section of skin tissue. Punch biopsies are ideal for obtaining both the epidermis and the upper layers of the dermis, making them useful for diagnosing conditions such as rashes, infections, and certain types of skin cancer.

2. Shave Biopsy: In this technique, a scalpel or a razor blade is used to shave off a superficial layer of the skin. Shave biopsies are primarily performed to diagnose skin lesions that are raised above the skin surface, such as moles or warts. These biopsies are relatively quick and straightforward, requiring no stitches.

3. Excisional Biopsy: When a deeper tissue sample is needed, an excisional biopsy is the preferred technique. It involves surgically removing the entire skin lesion or a significant portion of it. Excisional biopsies are commonly used to diagnose suspected melanomas or other types of skin cancer. The excised tissue is then sent to the laboratory for further analysis.

4. Incisional Biopsy: Unlike excisional biopsies, incisional biopsies involve the removal of only a small part of a larger skin lesion. This technique is employed when the entire lesion cannot be removed or when a representative sample is sufficient for diagnosis. Incisional biopsies are often used for large or deep lesions where removing the entire lesion might be impractical.

5. Frozen Section Biopsy: This type of biopsy is performed intraoperatively, mainly during surgical procedures for skin cancer. A thin layer of tissue is rapidly frozen and then examined under a microscope. Frozen section biopsies provide immediate results, allowing surgeons to make real-time decisions about the extent of tissue removal.

Understanding the different types of skin biopsies is essential for students pursuing a career in dermatology. Each biopsy technique has its indications and limitations, and choosing the appropriate method is crucial for accurate diagnosis and optimal patient care. By familiarizing themselves with these techniques, students will develop a solid foundation in dermatopathology, enabling them to provide accurate diagnoses and effective treatment plans in the future.

Specimen Collection and Handling

In the field of dermatopathology, the accurate collection and proper handling of specimens are of utmost importance. This subchapter will guide you, as students, on the essential steps and best practices for specimen collection and handling in dermatology.

1.   Introduction   to   Specimen   Collection: When dealing with dermatological conditions, it is crucial to obtain an appropriate sample that represents the lesion or affected area. This can be achieved through various methods, including biopsies, scrapings, swabs, and excisions. Each method has its own indications and specific techniques, which will be thoroughly explained in this chapter.

2.   Preparing   for   Specimen   Collection: Before collecting a specimen, it is vital to prepare yourself and the patient adequately. This involves explaining the procedure to the patient, obtaining informed consent, and ensuring a sterile environment. Proper preparation will not only ease the patient's anxiety but also yield better quality specimens for accurate diagnosis.

3.   Techniques   for   Specimen   Collection: This section will delve into the specific techniques used for various types of dermatological specimens. You will learn about punch biopsies, shave biopsies, excisions, scrapings, and swabs. The chapter will provide step-by-step instructions, including appropriate anesthesia, incision size, and the necessary tools for each technique.

4.   Handling   and   Transporting   Specimens: Once the specimen is collected, proper handling and transportation are crucial to preserve its integrity. This subchapter will guide you on

how to handle and process the specimens to ensure accurate diagnosis. Topics covered include specimen labeling, fixation, storage, and transportation methods, emphasizing the importance of timely processing to avoid specimen degradation.

5. Common Challenges and Troubleshooting: In dermatopathology, various challenges may arise during specimen collection and handling. This section will address some common issues such as inadequate sample size, improper fixation, contamination, and transport delays. Practical tips and troubleshooting strategies will be provided to help you overcome these challenges effectively.

6. Safety Precautions: Finally, this subchapter will emphasize the importance of safety precautions when handling dermatological specimens. It will cover topics such as personal protective equipment (PPE), proper disposal of sharps, and adherence to universal precautions to minimize the risk of infections and ensure a safe working environment.

By thoroughly understanding the principles and techniques of specimen collection and handling in dermatopathology, you will be equipped with the necessary skills to obtain accurate and reliable results. This subchapter serves as an essential guide for students in the field of dermatology, providing a solid foundation for your future practice in dermatopathology.

Important Considerations in Skin Specimen Processing

Skin specimen processing is a crucial step in dermatopathology, as it allows for accurate diagnosis and treatment of various skin conditions. As students in the field of dermatology, understanding the important considerations in skin specimen processing is vital for developing the necessary skills to become successful dermatopathologists. This subchapter aims to provide an overview of the key factors to consider when processing skin specimens, ensuring that students have a solid foundation in this essential aspect of dermatopathology.

The first consideration is proper handling and preservation of the skin specimen. Students must ensure that the specimen is handled delicately and preserved appropriately to prevent any damage or degradation. This involves correctly labeling the specimen, using appropriate containers, and maintaining the proper temperature during storage and transportation.

Secondly, it is crucial to consider the timing of processing skin specimens. Time is of the essence as delayed processing can result in tissue autolysis, which can affect the quality of the specimen and subsequent diagnosis. Students should be aware of the recommended time frame for processing different types of skin specimens and ensure they adhere to these guidelines.

Another important consideration is the selection of appropriate fixatives. Different fixatives have varying effects on tissue morphology and antigen preservation. Students should familiarize themselves with common fixatives used in dermatopathology, such as formalin and Michel's medium, and understand their advantages and limitations.

Furthermore, the choice of sectioning technique is crucial in skin specimen processing. Students should be proficient in using microtomes and cryostats to obtain thin, uniform sections for accurate diagnosis. Understanding the principles and techniques of different sectioning methods, such as routine paraffin sectioning and frozen sectioning, will greatly contribute to the quality of the processed skin specimen.

Lastly, the subchapter will discuss the importance of proper documentation and record-keeping during skin specimen processing. Accurate and detailed documentation of the specimen's origin, clinical history, and processing steps are essential for comprehensive dermatopathology reports. Students should develop good record-keeping habits to ensure that all necessary information is recorded accurately.

In conclusion, skin specimen processing is a critical aspect of dermatopathology that students in the field of dermatology must master. This subchapter provides an overview of important considerations in skin specimen processing, including proper handling and preservation, timing, selection of fixatives, sectioning techniques, and documentation. By understanding and implementing these considerations, students can ensure accurate diagnosis and contribute to the field of dermatopathology effectively.

Chapter 4: Dermatopathological Examination

Macroscopic Examination of Skin Specimens

In the field of dermatopathology, the macroscopic examination of skin specimens plays a vital role in the accurate diagnosis and treatment of dermatological conditions. This subchapter aims to provide students with a comprehensive understanding of the importance and techniques involved in macroscopic examination.

When analyzing skin specimens, dermatopathologists rely on macroscopic examination to gather initial information about the lesion or tissue sample. This examination involves careful observation of the specimen's color, size, shape, surface characteristics, and any additional features such as ulceration, scaling, or inflammation. By thoroughly examining these macroscopic features, students can begin to narrow down potential diagnoses and guide further microscopic analysis.

Color is an essential aspect of macroscopic examination, as it can provide valuable insights into the underlying pathology. For instance, a red or violaceous coloration may indicate inflammation, while a brown or black color may suggest melanocytic proliferation. Additionally, the size and shape of the lesion can help differentiate between various dermatological conditions, such as papules, plaques, nodules, or vesicles.

Surface characteristics, such as scaling, ulceration, or crusting, should be carefully noted during macroscopic examination. These features often provide clues about the underlying pathological process, such as psoriasis, squamous cell carcinoma, or infectious conditions like herpes simplex.

To ensure accurate macroscopic examination, students need to follow proper techniques. It is crucial to handle the specimen with care and avoid unnecessary manipulation or distortion. Adequate lighting and magnification tools should be used to enhance visibility and identify subtle features. Photographs may also be taken to document the macroscopic findings and aid in future reference.

In conclusion, macroscopic examination of skin specimens is a fundamental aspect of dermatopathology that allows students to gather initial information about the lesion or tissue sample. By carefully observing and documenting the color, size, shape, and surface characteristics of the specimen, students can begin to narrow down potential diagnoses and guide further microscopic analysis. Mastering the techniques involved in macroscopic examination is essential for accurate dermatological diagnoses and treatment planning.

Microscopic Examination of Skin Specimens

In the field of dermatology, microscopic examination of skin specimens is an essential diagnostic tool for dermatopathologists. This subchapter aims to introduce students to the principles and techniques involved in examining skin samples under a microscope.

To begin with, the collection of a skin specimen is crucial. It can be obtained through various methods such as shave biopsy, punch biopsy, or excisional biopsy, depending on the specific case. These specimens are subsequently fixed in formalin and processed for microscopic examination.

Once the skin specimen is properly prepared, it is sectioned into thin slices, usually around 4-6 micrometers thick. These sections are then mounted on glass slides and stained using special dyes, such as hematoxylin and eosin (H&E), which provide contrast and highlight different cellular structures.

Under the microscope, students will be able to observe the different layers of the skin, including the epidermis, dermis, and subcutaneous tissue. They will learn to identify various cell types, such as keratinocytes, melanocytes, and fibroblasts, as well as their specific features and distribution within the skin layers.

Furthermore, students will be introduced to the microscopic characteristics of different dermatological conditions. For example, they will learn to recognize the histopathological features of common skin diseases such as psoriasis, eczema, and skin cancers like melanoma and basal cell carcinoma. Through detailed descriptions and accompanying high-resolution images, students will gain a comprehensive understanding of the microscopic manifestations of these conditions.

In addition to the identification of specific cellular and tissue changes, students will also learn about the significance of immunohistochemistry (IHC) in dermatopathology. IHC allows for the detection of specific proteins or markers within the skin specimen, aiding in the diagnosis and classification of certain skin diseases.

Finally, students will be introduced to the concept of correlation between clinical and histopathological findings. By understanding the clinical presentation of a patient's skin condition and correlating it with microscopic examination, students will be able to develop a more accurate diagnosis and treatment plan.

In conclusion, the microscopic examination of skin specimens is a fundamental aspect of dermatopathology. By carefully studying the various cellular and tissue changes, students will acquire the skills necessary for accurate diagnosis and treatment of dermatological conditions. This subchapter provides a comprehensive overview of the techniques and principles involved in analyzing skin samples under the microscope, aimed at equipping students with the knowledge needed to excel in the field of dermatology.

Interpretation of Histopathology Reports

Histopathology reports are an essential component of dermatopathology, providing crucial information about the microscopic features of skin tissue specimens. As students in the field of dermatology, it is crucial to understand how to interpret these reports accurately. This subchapter will guide you through the process of interpreting histopathology reports, enabling you to gain a comprehensive understanding of the intricacies involved in this field.

Histopathology reports typically contain several sections that help in the interpretation of skin tissue samples. These sections include the clinical history, gross description, microscopic description, and diagnosis. Understanding each of these sections is pivotal for accurate interpretation.

The clinical history section provides important patient information, such as age, gender, and relevant medical history. It also includes details regarding the location and duration of the skin lesion, which can aid in narrowing down potential diagnoses.

The gross description section outlines the macroscopic appearance of the tissue sample, including its color, texture, and dimensions. This information is crucial as it helps to determine if any abnormalities are visible to the naked eye.

The microscopic description section is the most important part of the histopathology report. It details the microscopic features observed under the microscope, such as the presence of inflammatory cells, abnormal cell growth, and changes in tissue architecture. This section often includes the use of specific staining techniques to highlight certain components of the tissue.

The diagnosis section summarizes the findings from the microscopic examination and provides an overall diagnosis. It may include a specific disease or condition, or it may be more descriptive, such as "consistent with basal cell carcinoma."

To effectively interpret histopathology reports, students in dermatology must have a strong foundation in dermatopathology. This includes knowledge of different skin lesions, their histological features, and the corresponding clinical presentations. Regular exposure to a wide range of histopathology reports and attending dermatopathology conferences or workshops can help students to refine their skills in interpretation.

In conclusion, the interpretation of histopathology reports is a vital skill for students in dermatology. Understanding the different sections of a report, including clinical history, gross description, microscopic description, and diagnosis, is essential for accurate interpretation. Developing a strong foundation in dermatopathology and regularly practicing the interpretation of diverse histopathology reports will help students excel in this field.

Correlation of Clinical and Histopathological Findings

Understanding the correlation between clinical and histopathological findings is essential for students studying dermatopathology. Dermatology is a specialized field that deals with the diagnosis and treatment of skin disorders. Dermatopathology, on the other hand, focuses on the microscopic examination of skin tissues to identify and classify diseases.

When evaluating a skin lesion, dermatologists rely on both clinical and histopathological findings to arrive at an accurate diagnosis. Clinical findings include the patient's medical history, physical examination, and visual assessment of the lesion's appearance. Histopathological findings, on the other hand, involve the microscopic examination of a skin biopsy sample.

The correlation between clinical and histopathological findings plays a crucial role in dermatopathology. By correlating the two, students can develop the skills necessary to accurately diagnose various skin diseases. Here are some key aspects to consider:

1. Morphological Features: Clinical observations such as the size, shape, color, and texture of a skin lesion can provide valuable clues about its underlying histopathological characteristics. For example, a raised, erythematous lesion may indicate inflammation or an immune response, while a well-defined, pigmented lesion may suggest a benign neoplasm.

2. Differential Diagnosis: The correlation between clinical and histopathological findings helps in narrowing down the possible diagnoses. By examining the histopathological features of a skin

biopsy, students can confirm or rule out potential differential diagnoses suggested by the clinical presentation.

3. Treatment Planning: Accurate diagnosis is crucial for determining the appropriate treatment plan for a patient. By correlating clinical and histopathological findings, students can identify the specific disease process at play and select the most effective treatment options accordingly.

4. Communication: Effective communication between dermatologists and dermatopathologists is vital for accurate diagnosis and management of skin diseases. By understanding the correlation between clinical and histopathological findings, students can better communicate their observations and interpretations to ensure effective collaboration between these two specialties.

In conclusion, the correlation of clinical and histopathological findings is of utmost importance in dermatopathology. Students studying dermatology need to develop a comprehensive understanding of how to interpret both clinical and histopathological information in order to accurately diagnose and treat skin diseases. By mastering this correlation, students can provide optimal care to their patients and contribute to the field of dermatology.

Chapter 5: Inflammatory Skin Disorders

Acne Vulgaris

Acne vulgaris is a common skin condition that affects millions of people worldwide, particularly during adolescence. In this subchapter, we will delve into the intricacies of this condition, its causes, symptoms, and available treatment options. As students in the field of dermatology, it is crucial to have a comprehensive understanding of acne vulgaris as it is one of the most frequently encountered conditions in clinical practice.

Acne vulgaris, commonly referred to as acne, primarily affects the pilosebaceous units of the skin. These units consist of hair follicles and sebaceous glands, which produce sebum, an oily substance that keeps the skin moisturized. However, due to various factors such as hormonal imbalances, excess sebum production, and the colonization of the Propionibacterium acnes bacteria, the hair follicles become clogged, resulting in the formation of comedones, papules, pustules, nodules, or cysts.

The clinical presentation of acne vulgaris can vary from mild to severe, with symptoms including blackheads, whiteheads, red or inflamed bumps, and, in severe cases, painful nodules or cysts. Acne can significantly impact an individual's self-esteem and quality of life, making early diagnosis and effective treatment essential.

When it comes to treating acne vulgaris, a multifaceted approach is often necessary. This can include topical medications, such as retinoids, benzoyl peroxide, or antibiotics, which help reduce inflammation, unclog pores, and control bacterial overgrowth. In more severe cases, oral medications like isotretinoin may be prescribed to target the underlying causes of acne.

Additionally, lifestyle modifications, such as practicing good hygiene, avoiding excessive scrubbing or squeezing of lesions, and adopting a healthy diet, can also play a significant role in managing acne vulgaris. It is crucial for students to educate their patients about the importance of these lifestyle changes alongside medical interventions.

In conclusion, acne vulgaris is a prevalent dermatological condition that requires a holistic approach for effective management. By understanding the pathogenesis, clinical presentation, and treatment options available, students in dermatology can provide comprehensive care to their patients. Acne vulgaris can have a lasting impact on an individual's physical and emotional well-being, underscoring the importance of early intervention and ongoing education in the field of dermatopathology.

Psoriasis

Psoriasis: Understanding and Managing a Chronic Skin Condition

Psoriasis is a chronic skin disorder that affects millions of people worldwide. It is an autoimmune disease characterized by the rapid turnover of skin cells, resulting in the formation of thick, red, and scaly patches on the skin. This condition can significantly impact a person's quality of life, causing physical discomfort and emotional distress. In this subchapter, we will explore the various aspects of psoriasis, including its causes, symptoms, diagnosis, and management strategies.

Causes of Psoriasis: While the exact cause of psoriasis remains unknown, it is believed to result from a combination of genetic and environmental factors. Certain genes are thought to play a role in the development of psoriasis, and triggers such as stress, infections, and certain medications can exacerbate the condition.

Symptoms and Clinical Presentation: Psoriasis primarily affects the skin, with characteristic symptoms including raised, inflamed patches covered with silvery scales. These patches commonly appear on the elbows, knees, scalp, and lower back, but can also affect other areas of the body. The severity of symptoms can vary widely among individuals, with some experiencing mild discomfort while others face debilitating symptoms.

Diagnosis of Psoriasis: Diagnosing psoriasis involves a thorough examination of the affected skin and medical history evaluation. Dermatologists may also perform a skin biopsy to confirm the diagnosis and rule out other similar skin conditions. Understanding the different clinical variants of psoriasis, such as plaque psoriasis, guttate psoriasis, and pustular psoriasis, is crucial for accurate diagnosis and treatment.

Management   Strategies:
While psoriasis is a chronic condition without a known cure, there are several effective management strategies available to alleviate symptoms and improve quality of life. Treatment options may include topical medications, phototherapy, systemic medications, and biologic agents. Dermatologists often tailor treatment plans to suit individual needs, considering factors such as severity, location, and patient preferences.

Living   with   Psoriasis:
Psoriasis not only affects the physical health of individuals but also poses emotional and psychological challenges. Students pursuing dermatology must be aware of the impact that psoriasis can have on patients' mental health and well-being. Providing support, education, and counseling to patients can help them cope with the challenges associated with this chronic condition.

Conclusion:
Psoriasis is a complex and chronic skin condition that demands comprehensive understanding and management. As students in the field of dermatology, it is crucial to be well-versed in the causes, symptoms, diagnosis, and treatment options for psoriasis. By staying updated with the latest research and advancements, students can contribute to the development of innovative strategies to improve the lives of individuals living with psoriasis.

Eczematous Dermatitis

Eczematous dermatitis is a common skin condition characterized by inflammation, redness, itching, and the formation of small fluid-filled blisters. It is a type of dermatitis that primarily affects the epidermis, the outermost layer of the skin. This subchapter will provide a comprehensive overview of eczematous dermatitis, including its causes, symptoms, diagnosis, and treatment options.

Causes:

Eczematous dermatitis can be caused by a variety of factors, including genetic predisposition, allergies, irritants, and environmental triggers. Individuals with a family history of eczema or atopic diseases are more likely to develop eczematous dermatitis. Common triggers include certain foods, pollen, dust mites, pet dander, and exposure to harsh chemicals or fabrics.

Symptoms:

The main symptom of eczematous dermatitis is intense itching, which can lead to scratching and subsequent skin damage. This can result in a vicious cycle of itching and scratching, causing the affected area to become red, swollen, and crusted. In some cases, small fluid-filled blisters may form, which can then rupture and ooze. The most commonly affected areas include the hands, feet, face, and flexural areas such as the elbows and knees.

Diagnosis:

Diagnosing eczematous dermatitis involves a thorough physical examination and a detailed medical history. The dermatologist may ask about the patient's symptoms, triggers, and family history of eczema or other skin conditions. In some cases, additional tests such as patch testing or blood tests may be recommended to identify specific allergens or underlying conditions.

Treatment:

The treatment of eczematous dermatitis aims to relieve symptoms, reduce inflammation, and prevent flare-ups. This may involve the use of topical corticosteroids, which help reduce inflammation and itching. Moisturizers and emollients are also essential to keep the skin hydrated and prevent dryness. Additionally, identifying and avoiding triggers is crucial to managing the condition. In severe cases, oral medications or phototherapy may be prescribed.

Prevention:

Preventing eczematous dermatitis involves avoiding known triggers and maintaining good skin care practices. This includes using gentle cleansers, avoiding harsh soaps or detergents, and moisturizing the skin regularly. It is also important to wear protective clothing, such as gloves or long sleeves, when exposed to irritants or allergens.

In conclusion, eczematous dermatitis is a common inflammatory skin condition that can significantly impact an individual's quality of life. Understanding its causes, symptoms, and treatment options can help students gain valuable knowledge in the field of dermatology. By recognizing and managing eczematous dermatitis effectively, healthcare professionals can provide optimal care and improve the overall well-being of their patients.

Lichen Planus

Introduction:

Lichen planus is a chronic inflammatory condition that affects the skin, mucous membranes, hair, and nails. It is a common dermatological disorder encountered in clinical practice, with a prevalence of approximately 1-2% in the general population. This subchapter aims to provide students with a comprehensive understanding of lichen planus, including its etiology, clinical presentation, histopathology, and management.

Etiology:

The exact cause of lichen planus remains unknown; however, several factors contribute to its development. These may include genetic predisposition, autoimmune mechanisms, viral infections (such as hepatitis C), certain medications, and environmental triggers. It is essential for students to be aware of these factors to better understand the pathogenesis of the disease.

Clinical Presentation:

Lichen planus typically presents as pruritic, polygonal, violaceous papules or plaques that can occur anywhere on the body. The lesions may be flat or raised and often exhibit a distinctive "Wickham's striae" pattern, which appears as white, lacy lines on the surface. Students should be familiar with the various clinical variants of lichen planus, such as hypertrophic, erosive, and bullous forms, as well as the involvement of mucous membranes, scalp, and nails.

Histopathology:

Histopathological examination is crucial for the diagnosis of lichen planus. Students should become familiar with the characteristic findings, which include hyperkeratosis, irregular acanthosis, sawtooth rete ridges, and a dense band-like lymphocytic infiltrate in the upper dermis. The presence of Civatte bodies, which are degenerated basal cells, is also a hallmark feature. Understanding these histopathological features will enable students to differentiate lichen planus from other similar dermatoses.

Management:

The management of lichen planus involves both symptomatic relief and disease control. Topical corticosteroids are the mainstay of treatment for localized disease, while oral corticosteroids or immunosuppressive agents may be necessary for widespread or severe cases. Students should also be aware of the potential complications associated with lichen planus, such as secondary infection, scarring, and the increased risk of squamous cell carcinoma in long-standing cases.

Conclusion:

Lichen planus is a common dermatological condition that requires a thorough understanding for accurate diagnosis and appropriate management. By familiarizing themselves with the etiology, clinical presentation, histopathology, and treatment options, students will be better equipped to recognize and manage this challenging disease in their future dermatology practice.

Vasculitis

Vasculitis is a complex and fascinating topic within the field of dermatology. It refers to a group of conditions characterized by inflammation of blood vessels, which can have significant implications for the skin and other organs. Understanding the various types of vasculitis and their clinical presentation is essential for dermatology students.

One of the most common types of vasculitis is called cutaneous small vessel vasculitis (CSVV). This condition primarily affects the small blood vessels in the skin, resulting in palpable purpura, or small raised purple spots. CSVV can be caused by infections, medications, or systemic diseases such as rheumatoid arthritis or lupus. Recognizing the characteristic skin findings and understanding the underlying causes are crucial for accurate diagnosis and management.

Another important type of vasculitis is known as leukocytoclastic vasculitis (LCV). This condition is characterized by inflammation of the small blood vessels caused by the deposition of immune complexes. LCV typically presents as palpable purpura and can be associated with infections, medications, or underlying systemic diseases. Dermatology students need to be familiar with the histopathological features of LCV, which include leukocytoclasia, or the destruction of white blood cells within blood vessel walls.

In addition to CSVV and LCV, there are several other types of vasculitis that dermatology students should be aware of. These include medium vessel vasculitis, such as polyarteritis nodosa, and large vessel vasculitis, such as giant cell arteritis. Each type has its unique clinical presentation, associated systemic manifestations, and histopathological features.

Accurate diagnosis of vasculitis requires a combination of clinical, histopathological, and laboratory findings. Dermatology students should be familiar with the diagnostic criteria for different types of vasculitis and understand the role of skin biopsies in confirming the diagnosis.

Treatment of vasculitis involves a multidisciplinary approach, often involving rheumatologists and other specialists. Immunosuppressive medications, such as corticosteroids and disease-modifying antirheumatic drugs, are commonly used to control inflammation and prevent organ damage.

In conclusion, vasculitis is a challenging yet fascinating topic within dermatology. Familiarizing oneself with the various types, clinical presentations, and diagnostic approaches is essential for dermatology students. By understanding vasculitis, students can provide accurate diagnoses and appropriate management, ultimately improving patient outcomes.

Chapter 6: Infectious Skin Conditions

Bacterial Infections

In the field of dermatology, understanding bacterial infections is crucial for students to effectively diagnose and treat various skin conditions. Bacterial infections are among the most common and widespread skin ailments encountered by dermatologists. This subchapter will provide students with a comprehensive overview of bacterial infections, including their causes, symptoms, and treatment options.

Causes:
Bacterial infections occur when harmful bacteria invade the skin, causing an inflammatory response. The most common bacteria responsible for skin infections include Staphylococcus aureus and Streptococcus pyogenes. These bacteria can enter the skin through cuts, wounds, or hair follicles, leading to infections such as impetigo, cellulitis, and folliculitis.

Symptoms:
The symptoms of bacterial infections vary depending on the type and severity of the infection. Common signs include redness, swelling, warmth, and pain in the affected area. Pus or discharge may also be present in some cases. Additionally, bacterial infections can cause systemic symptoms like fever and malaise.

Types:
Students should familiarize themselves with different types of bacterial infections commonly encountered in dermatology. Impetigo, a highly

contagious infection, is characterized by honey-colored crusts and fluid-filled blisters. Cellulitis, on the other hand, is a deeper infection that causes redness, swelling, and tenderness. Folliculitis affects the hair follicles, leading to small, red bumps or pustules.

Treatment:
Prompt and appropriate treatment is essential to manage bacterial infections effectively. Treatment options may include topical or oral antibiotics, depending on the severity of the infection. In some cases, incision and drainage of abscesses or surgical debridement may be necessary. It is important for students to understand the indications, contraindications, and potential side effects of various treatment modalities.

Prevention:
Preventing bacterial infections is crucial to maintain good skin health. Students should learn about preventive measures, including proper wound care, regular hand hygiene, and avoiding sharing personal items. Vaccinations against certain bacteria, such as tetanus and pneumococcus, can also help prevent infections.

In conclusion, bacterial infections are a common and significant aspect of dermatology that students must be well-versed in. By understanding the causes, symptoms, types, treatment options, and preventive measures of bacterial infections, students can develop the necessary skills to diagnose and manage these conditions effectively. Continual learning and staying updated with the latest research and guidelines will further enhance students' ability to provide optimal care for patients with bacterial infections.

Viral Infections

In the field of dermatology, one of the significant areas of concern is viral infections. These infections are caused by viruses that can invade the skin and mucous membranes, leading to a wide range of dermatological conditions. Understanding viral infections is crucial for students studying dermatopathology, as it helps in the diagnosis, treatment, and prevention of these conditions.

One of the most common viral infections encountered in dermatology is herpes simplex. This viral infection presents as clustered vesicles or blisters on the skin and is caused by the herpes simplex virus (HSV). Herpes simplex can be categorized into two types: HSV-1, which primarily affects the oral area, and HSV-2, which is responsible for genital herpes. Students should be aware of the clinical presentation, diagnostic tests, and management options for herpes simplex infections.

Another viral infection of concern is human papillomavirus (HPV). HPV infection can lead to the development of warts, particularly on the hands, feet, and genital area. Understanding the different types of HPV strains and their associated clinical manifestations is essential for the accurate diagnosis and treatment of these infections.

Furthermore, students should be familiar with viral exanthems, which are skin rashes caused by viral infections. These rashes can be seen in various viral illnesses such as measles, rubella, and chickenpox. Recognizing the characteristic patterns of these exanthems is vital for early identification and appropriate management.

In addition to these common viral infections, students should also learn about less frequently encountered viral conditions such as molluscum contagiosum, viral hemorrhagic fevers, and viral exanthems in immunocompromised individuals. Understanding the pathogenesis, clinical features, and diagnostic methods for these viral infections will contribute to a comprehensive understanding of dermatopathology.

Prevention plays a significant role in managing viral infections. Students should be educated about vaccination strategies and the importance of public health measures in preventing the spread of viral infections. Additionally, understanding the role of antiviral medications in the treatment of specific viral infections is essential for students pursuing a career in dermatology.

In conclusion, the subchapter on viral infections in "The Complete Guide to Dermatopathology for Students" provides a comprehensive overview of the various viral infections encountered in dermatology. By familiarizing themselves with the clinical presentations, diagnostic methods, and management options for viral infections, students will develop the necessary skills to effectively diagnose and treat these conditions. Furthermore, understanding the preventive measures and vaccination strategies will contribute to their overall knowledge in the field of dermatology, equipping them to provide optimal care to their patients.

Fungal Infections

Fungal infections are a common dermatological concern that affects individuals of all ages and backgrounds. In this subchapter, we will delve into the world of fungal infections, exploring their causes, symptoms, diagnosis, and treatment options. Whether you are a medical student or a budding dermatologist, this comprehensive guide will equip you with the knowledge needed to identify and manage these conditions effectively.

Fungi are microorganisms that can be found in various environments, including soil, plants, and even on our own bodies. While most fungi are harmless, some can cause infections when they penetrate the skin, hair, or nails. These infections can present in various forms, such as ringworm, athlete's foot, or nail fungus.

Understanding the signs and symptoms of fungal infections is crucial for accurate diagnosis. Patients may experience redness, itching, scaling, or the formation of blisters or pustules. These symptoms can vary depending on the type of infection and the affected area. It is essential to differentiate between fungal infections and other dermatological conditions to provide appropriate treatment.

Diagnosing a fungal infection often involves a combination of clinical examination, medical history assessment, and laboratory tests. Dermatopathologists may collect skin or nail samples for microscopic examination, utilizing techniques such as potassium hydroxide (KOH) testing or fungal cultures. Accurate diagnosis is essential for tailoring the most effective treatment plan.

Treatment options for fungal infections typically involve the use of antifungal medications. Topical creams, powders, or ointments are commonly prescribed for superficial infections, while oral antifungal medications are reserved for more severe or systemic cases. It is crucial to educate patients about the importance of good hygiene practices and the prevention of reinfection.

Furthermore, this subchapter will explore some of the common risk factors for fungal infections, including compromised immune systems, excessive sweating, poor hygiene, and close contact with infected individuals. By understanding these risk factors, students can develop a comprehensive approach to patient care and preventive measures.

In conclusion, fungal infections are prevalent in dermatology and require proper identification and management. This subchapter provides students with a comprehensive understanding of fungal infections, including their causes, symptoms, diagnosis, and treatment options. By equipping students with this knowledge, they will be better prepared to diagnose and treat fungal infections effectively, ensuring optimal patient care in the field of dermatology.

Parasitic Infections

Parasitic infections represent a significant aspect of dermatology that students must familiarize themselves with in order to provide comprehensive patient care. This subchapter explores the various types of parasitic infections that can affect the skin, their clinical presentations, diagnostic methods, and treatment options.

Introduction:
Parasitic infections are caused by organisms that live at the expense of their host, taking vital nutrients and causing damage to the skin and other tissues. In dermatology, several parasitic infections can present with distinct clinical features, making their identification crucial for accurate diagnosis and management.

Key Types of Parasitic Infections:

1. Scabies: This highly contagious infestation is caused by the Sarcoptes scabiei mite. Students will learn about the characteristic burrows, intense itching, and diagnostic techniques such as skin scraping.

2. Pediculosis: Pediculosis, commonly known as lice infestation, involves the head, body, or pubic area. Students will understand the various types of lice, their clinical presentations, and treatment options.

3. Cutaneous larva migrans: This condition occurs when larvae of certain parasites, such as hookworms, penetrate the skin, causing an itchy and serpiginous rash. Students will explore the epidemiology, clinical features, and management of this condition.

4. Leishmaniasis: Focusing on the cutaneous form of leishmaniasis, this section covers the causative agent, transmission, clinical manifestations, and diagnostic methods for this parasitic infection.

Diagnosis and Management: Students will be introduced to the diagnostic tools commonly used in dermatopathology for identifying parasitic infections, including microscopy, skin biopsies, and serological tests. Treatment options, such as topical medications, oral antiparasitic drugs, and environmental hygiene, will also be discussed.

Prevention and Public Health: Understanding the preventive measures against parasitic infections is essential for students to educate patients and contribute to public health initiatives. This section delves into strategies for prevention, including personal hygiene, environmental sanitation, and public health education.

Conclusion:
Parasitic infections are a significant component of dermatopathology, and students must be equipped with the knowledge and skills to identify, diagnose, and manage these conditions effectively. By understanding the various types of parasitic infections, their clinical presentations, diagnostic methods, and treatment options, students will be better prepared to provide comprehensive care to their patients and contribute to the field of dermatology.

Chapter 7: Neoplastic Skin Conditions

Benign Skin Tumors

In the vast field of dermatology, the study of skin tumors holds significant importance. Dermatopathology, a specialized branch of dermatology, focuses on the examination and diagnosis of skin diseases and tumors. One crucial aspect of dermatopathology is the understanding of benign skin tumors.

Benign skin tumors are non-cancerous growths that arise from the skin layers. Although they do not pose a threat to health, they can still cause discomfort and affect a patient's quality of life. As students diving into the world of dermatopathology, it is essential to familiarize ourselves with the various types and characteristics of benign skin tumors.

One of the most common benign skin tumors is the seborrheic keratosis. These growths typically appear as raised, waxy, and pigmented lesions on the skin. Although they may resemble melanoma, seborrheic keratosis can be easily differentiated through clinical and histopathological examination.

Another type of benign skin tumor is the epidermal inclusion cyst. These cysts are formed when a hair follicle becomes blocked, leading to the accumulation of keratin within the skin. Epidermal inclusion cysts are typically round, firm, and painless. Understanding their distinct features is crucial to avoid misdiagnosis and unnecessary procedures.

Fibroepithelial polyps, also known as skin tags, are another common benign skin tumor encountered in dermatopathology. These soft, pedunculated growths often occur in areas of friction, such as the neck, underarms, and groin. While they are harmless, patients may seek their removal for cosmetic purposes.

Dermatofibromas, on the other hand, present as firm, brownish nodules on the skin. These benign tumors result from the proliferation of fibroblasts, and their exact cause remains unknown. Dermatofibromas can be easily diagnosed through clinical examination and histopathological evaluation.

Lastly, the pilomatricoma is a benign skin tumor that arises from the hair matrix cells. These slow-growing tumors typically appear as firm, solitary nodules, often on the face or upper extremities. Pilomatricomas are commonly seen in children and adolescents, and their diagnosis can be confirmed through histopathological examination.

As students delving into dermatopathology, it is crucial to recognize and differentiate between various benign skin tumors. Through comprehensive understanding, we can ensure accurate diagnoses, provide appropriate treatment options, and alleviate any concerns our patients may have. By mastering the knowledge of benign skin tumors, we lay a strong foundation for our future careers in dermatology and dermatopathology.

Premalignant Skin Lesions

In the world of dermatology, premalignant skin lesions are a topic of significant importance. These lesions are characterized by their potential to progress into skin cancer if left untreated. As students exploring the field of dermatopathology, it is crucial to have a comprehensive understanding of these lesions to effectively diagnose and manage them.

Premalignant skin lesions encompass a range of conditions, including actinic keratosis, Bowen's disease, and lentigo maligna. Actinic keratosis, also known as solar keratosis, is one of the most common premalignant lesions. It typically appears as rough, scaly patches on sun-exposed areas such as the face, scalp, and hands. If left untreated, actinic keratosis can transform into squamous cell carcinoma.

Bowen's disease, on the other hand, presents as well-demarcated, erythematous patches with a scaly surface. These lesions are most commonly found on the lower extremities, but they can occur in other areas as well. Bowen's disease is considered an early form of squamous cell carcinoma and should be closely monitored and treated accordingly.

Lentigo maligna, often seen in older individuals with a history of sun exposure, manifests as irregular pigmented patches on sun-exposed areas, particularly the face. This lesion has the potential to progress to lentigo maligna melanoma, a highly invasive and aggressive form of skin cancer. Early detection and intervention are key in preventing its progression.

Diagnosing premalignant skin lesions involves a combination of clinical evaluation and histopathological examination. Students should familiarize themselves with the clinical characteristics, such as size, shape, color, and texture, as well as any associated symptoms. Histopathological examination, through skin biopsies, allows for a more accurate diagnosis by assessing the cellular changes within the lesion.

Management of premalignant skin lesions primarily revolves around their removal or destruction. This can be achieved through various methods, including cryotherapy, topical medications, photodynamic therapy, and surgical excision. The choice of treatment depends on factors such as lesion size, location, and patient preference. Regular follow-up examinations are essential to monitor the lesions and ensure they do not progress or recur.

As future dermatopathologists, it is crucial for students to understand premalignant skin lesions thoroughly. Recognizing their clinical presentation, accurately diagnosing through histopathological examination, and implementing appropriate management strategies are vital in preventing the progression to skin cancer. By gaining expertise in this area, students can make significant contributions to the field of dermatology and positively impact patient outcomes.

Skin Cancer

Skin cancer is a significant concern in the field of dermatology. As future dermatologists, it is crucial for students to have a comprehensive understanding of this malignant condition. This subchapter aims to provide students with an overview of skin cancer, including its types, causes, risk factors, diagnosis, and treatment options.

Skin cancer is the abnormal growth of skin cells, primarily caused by prolonged exposure to ultraviolet (UV) radiation from the sun or artificial sources such as tanning beds. The most common types of skin cancer are basal cell carcinoma, squamous cell carcinoma, and melanoma. Basal cell carcinoma and squamous cell carcinoma are generally less aggressive and have a high cure rate when detected and treated early. On the other hand, melanoma is the most dangerous type of skin cancer, with the potential to spread to other parts of the body.

Several risk factors increase the likelihood of developing skin cancer. These include fair skin, a history of sunburns, excessive sun exposure, a family history of skin cancer, a weakened immune system, and the presence of certain genetic conditions. It is important for students to educate themselves and their patients about these risk factors to promote early detection and prevention.

Detecting skin cancer involves a thorough examination of the skin, including the use of dermatoscopy and biopsies for suspicious lesions. Students will learn about the ABCDE rule, which provides guidelines for identifying potential melanomas based on asymmetry, border irregularity, color variation, diameter, and evolution of lesions. Early diagnosis significantly improves the prognosis and treatment outcomes for patients.

Treatment options for skin cancer depend on various factors, such as the type, location, and stage of the cancer. Some common treatment modalities include surgical excision, cryosurgery, radiation therapy, topical medications, and chemotherapy. Students will gain insights into the indications, benefits, and potential risks associated with each treatment option.

In conclusion, this subchapter on skin cancer provides students with essential knowledge about the types, causes, risk factors, diagnosis, and treatment options for this prevalent dermatological condition. By equipping themselves with this information, students will be better prepared to diagnose, treat, and educate their patients about skin cancer, ultimately contributing to the prevention and early detection of this potentially life-threatening disease.

Melanocytic Lesions

Melanocytic lesions are a diverse group of skin conditions that involve the proliferation of melanocytes, the cells responsible for producing melanin, the pigment that gives color to our skin, hair, and eyes. These lesions can range from benign moles to potentially malignant melanomas, making their accurate diagnosis crucial in the field of dermatology.

Understanding the various types of melanocytic lesions is essential for dermatology students, as it enables them to differentiate between benign and malignant lesions and determine appropriate treatment plans for their patients. This subchapter will provide an overview of the common melanocytic lesions encountered in clinical practice and the key features that aid in their diagnosis.

One of the most common benign melanocytic lesions is the common mole, also known as a melanocytic nevus. These lesions typically appear as small, well-defined, pigmented macules or papules on the skin. Students will learn about the different types of melanocytic nevi, such as junctional, compound, and dermal nevi, and the characteristic histological features that distinguish them.

Another important topic covered in this subchapter is dysplastic nevi, also known as atypical moles. These lesions are larger and have an irregular shape, color, and border. Students will learn how to recognize the clinical and histological features of dysplastic nevi and understand their significance as potential precursors to melanoma.

Furthermore, the subchapter will delve into the diagnosis and management of melanoma, the most aggressive form of skin cancer.

Students will be introduced to the ABCDE (asymmetry, border irregularity, color variation, diameter greater than 6 mm, and evolving) mnemonic for recognizing suspicious melanocytic lesions. They will also learn about the different subtypes of melanoma, including superficial spreading melanoma, nodular melanoma, and lentigo maligna melanoma, and the histological characteristics that aid in their diagnosis.

To enhance learning, this subchapter will include high-quality clinical and histopathological images of melanocytic lesions, allowing students to develop their visual recognition skills. Additionally, case studies and interactive quizzes will be provided to test students' understanding and reinforce key concepts.

By the end of this subchapter, students will have acquired a solid foundation in the identification and characterization of melanocytic lesions. This knowledge will empower them to make accurate diagnoses, provide appropriate treatment options, and effectively communicate with patients about their condition.

Cutaneous Lymphomas

Lymphomas are a type of cancer that originate in the lymphatic system, which is responsible for carrying immune cells throughout the body. When lymphomas develop in the skin, they are referred to as cutaneous lymphomas. This subchapter aims to provide students in the field of dermatology with a comprehensive understanding of cutaneous lymphomas, their classification, diagnostic techniques, and treatment options.

Classification:
Cutaneous lymphomas can be broadly classified into two main categories: primary cutaneous lymphomas and secondary cutaneous involvement in systemic lymphomas. Primary cutaneous lymphomas primarily involve the skin and have a distinct clinical and histological presentation. Secondary cutaneous involvement occurs when lymphoma cells spread from other organs or systems to the skin.

Diagnostic   Techniques:
Accurate diagnosis of cutaneous lymphomas requires a multidisciplinary approach. Dermatologists, pathologists, and oncologists collaborate to gather clinical information, perform skin biopsies, and analyze laboratory findings. Histopathological examination of skin samples, immunohistochemistry, and molecular studies play a crucial role in distinguishing different subtypes of cutaneous lymphomas.

Common   Subtypes:
The most common subtypes of cutaneous lymphomas include mycosis fungoides (MF) and Sézary syndrome (SS). MF usually presents as a

chronic, itchy, and scaly rash that mimics eczema. SS, on the other hand, is an aggressive form of cutaneous lymphoma characterized by erythroderma, lymphadenopathy, and circulating malignant T-cells.

Treatment Options:
Treatment strategies for cutaneous lymphomas depend on various factors such as disease stage, subtype, and patient characteristics. Localized disease may be managed with topical therapies, phototherapy, or radiation. Systemic treatments, such as chemotherapy, immunotherapy, and targeted therapies, are often used for advanced or disseminated cutaneous lymphomas. Multidisciplinary care, including regular follow-ups and supportive care, is crucial for optimizing patient outcomes.

Future Directions:
Advancements in molecular and genetic techniques have enabled researchers to identify distinct molecular profiles and genetic alterations in cutaneous lymphomas. This knowledge has led to the development of targeted therapies and immunotherapies, providing new treatment options with improved efficacy and reduced side effects. Additionally, ongoing clinical trials are exploring novel therapeutic approaches, and students should stay updated with the latest research in this rapidly evolving field.

In conclusion, understanding cutaneous lymphomas is essential for students pursuing a career in dermatology. By familiarizing themselves with the classification, diagnostic techniques, and treatment options, students can contribute to the early detection, accurate diagnosis, and optimal management of cutaneous lymphomas, ultimately improving patient outcomes.

Chapter 8: Autoimmune and Connective Tissue Disorders

Systemic Lupus Erythematosus

Systemic Lupus Erythematosus (SLE) is a chronic autoimmune disease that predominantly affects women of childbearing age. It is a multisystem disorder characterized by the production of autoantibodies, immune complex deposition, and subsequent inflammation in various organs, including the skin.

Skin involvement is common in SLE and can manifest in different ways. The classic cutaneous finding is the "butterfly rash," also known as malar erythema, which appears as a symmetrical, erythematous rash across the cheeks and bridge of the nose. Other skin manifestations include discoid lupus erythematosus (DLE), subacute cutaneous lupus erythematosus (SCLE), and vasculitis. It is crucial for dermatologists to recognize these skin lesions, as they can be the first sign of systemic disease and help guide further diagnostic workup.

DLE is characterized by the presence of well-defined, erythematous plaques with adherent scales and follicular plugging. These lesions typically occur on sun-exposed areas, such as the face, scalp, and ears. Over time, they can lead to scarring and permanent hair loss. Histopathological examination of lesional skin reveals hyperkeratosis, follicular plugging, and a dense inflammatory infiltrate in the dermis, composed of lymphocytes, plasma cells, and histiocytes.

SCLE presents as annular, psoriasiform, or papulosquamous lesions that are usually photosensitive. They are most commonly found on the upper trunk, neck, and arms. Histopathological examination shows interface dermatitis with vacuolar degeneration of the basal layer, apoptotic keratinocytes, and a perivascular lymphocytic infiltrate.

Vasculitis in SLE can manifest as palpable purpura, ulcers, or livedo reticularis. Histopathological examination may reveal leukocytoclastic vasculitis with neutrophilic infiltration around blood vessels.

In addition to skin involvement, SLE can affect multiple organs, including the kidneys, heart, lungs, and joints. It is important for dermatopathology students to be aware of these systemic manifestations and their potential impact on patient management.

Diagnosis of SLE is based on clinical and laboratory findings, including the presence of antinuclear antibodies (ANA) and other autoantibodies. Treatment involves a multidisciplinary approach with nonsteroidal anti-inflammatory drugs (NSAIDs), corticosteroids, immunosuppressants, and hydroxychloroquine.

In conclusion, SLE is a complex autoimmune disease with a wide range of cutaneous manifestations. Dermatologists play a crucial role in recognizing and diagnosing these skin lesions, which can be the initial clue to the presence of systemic disease. It is essential for dermatopathology students to familiarize themselves with the various skin findings associated with SLE and understand the importance of a multidisciplinary approach for optimal patient care.

Dermatomyositis

Dermatomyositis is a rare autoimmune disease that primarily affects the skin and muscles. In this subchapter, we will explore the key aspects of dermatomyositis, including its etiology, clinical presentation, diagnostic testing, and treatment options. This information is specifically tailored for students in the field of dermatology, who are seeking a comprehensive understanding of this condition.

Dermatomyositis is characterized by inflammation of the skin and underlying muscles, resulting in characteristic skin findings and muscle weakness. The exact cause of this disease remains unknown, although it is thought to involve a combination of genetic predisposition and environmental triggers. It is more commonly observed in children and adults between the ages of 40 and 60.

Clinical manifestations of dermatomyositis include a distinct skin rash, often referred to as the "heliotrope rash," which appears as a purplish discoloration around the eyes. Other common skin findings include Gottron's papules, which are raised patches on the knuckles, elbows, and knees, and the "shawl sign," which presents as a red or purple rash on the upper back and shoulders. Muscle weakness is usually symmetric and can affect both proximal and distal muscle groups.

Diagnosis of dermatomyositis involves a combination of clinical examination, laboratory testing, and histopathological analysis. Blood tests may reveal elevated levels of muscle enzymes, such as creatine kinase (CK), and autoantibodies, including anti-Jo-1 and anti-Mi-2. A muscle biopsy is often performed to confirm the diagnosis and evaluate the extent of muscle inflammation.

Treatment strategies for dermatomyositis aim to control inflammation, alleviate symptoms, and prevent complications. This typically involves the use of corticosteroids, such as prednisone, to suppress the immune response. Immunosuppressive drugs, such as methotrexate or azathioprine, may be added for more severe or refractory cases. Physical therapy and exercise programs are crucial for maintaining muscle strength and function.

In summary, dermatomyositis is an autoimmune disease that primarily affects the skin and muscles. Its clinical presentation and diagnostic testing are essential for accurate diagnosis and appropriate management. By understanding the etiology, clinical features, and treatment options of dermatomyositis, students in the field of dermatology can better identify and manage this complex condition.

Scleroderma

Scleroderma is a rare and complex autoimmune disease that primarily affects the skin, but can also involve other organs such as the lungs, heart, kidneys, and gastrointestinal tract. In this subchapter, we will explore the clinical and histopathological aspects of scleroderma, providing students with a comprehensive understanding of this condition within the field of dermatology.

Clinical   Features:
Scleroderma presents with a wide range of clinical features, which can vary from patient to patient. The hallmark of this condition is the excessive production and deposition of collagen in the skin and other affected organs. As a result, patients often experience thickening and hardening of the skin, especially on the extremities and face. This can lead to limited mobility and joint stiffness. Other common symptoms include Raynaud's phenomenon, where the fingers and toes turn white or blue in response to cold temperatures or stress, and digital ulcers. Internal organ involvement may manifest as difficulty swallowing, shortness of breath, or compromised kidney function.

Histopathological   Findings:
To establish a definitive diagnosis of scleroderma, a skin biopsy is often performed. Histopathological examination of affected skin reveals characteristic findings. The epidermis may show atrophy, thinning, or hyperkeratosis. The dermis exhibits increased collagen deposition, resulting in a thickened and homogenized appearance. This is known as "sclerosis." The collagen bundles may extend deeper into the subcutaneous tissue, affecting the adnexal structures such as

hair follicles and sweat glands. In some cases, a perivascular lymphocytic infiltrate can be observed.

Treatment and Management: Scleroderma is a chronic condition with no known cure. However, various treatment options are available to manage symptoms and slow disease progression. Pharmacological interventions, such as immunosuppressive agents, can help reduce inflammation and control autoimmune responses. Physical therapy and regular exercise are crucial to maintain joint mobility and prevent contractures. Additionally, patients are advised to protect their skin from extreme temperatures, wear appropriate clothing, and use moisturizers to alleviate dryness.

Conclusion:
Scleroderma is a complex autoimmune disease that primarily affects the skin but can also involve other organs. Understanding the clinical and histopathological aspects of this condition is essential for students studying dermatopathology. By recognizing the characteristic features of scleroderma, students will be better equipped to diagnose and manage this challenging disease within the field of dermatology.

Bullous Diseases

Bullous diseases are a group of dermatological conditions characterized by the formation of fluid-filled blisters on the skin. These blisters can vary in size and may be accompanied by other symptoms such as itching, pain, or inflammation. Understanding the different types of bullous diseases is crucial for students in the field of dermatology, as it allows for accurate diagnosis and appropriate treatment.

1. Pemphigus: Pemphigus is an autoimmune blistering disorder that affects the skin and mucous membranes. It is characterized by the formation of fragile blisters that easily rupture, leaving behind erosions. There are several subtypes of pemphigus, including pemphigus vulgaris and pemphigus foliaceus, each with distinct clinical and histological features.

2. Bullous pemphigoid: Bullous pemphigoid is another autoimmune blistering disorder that predominantly affects the elderly. It is characterized by the formation of large, tense blisters on the skin. Unlike pemphigus, bullous pemphigoid blisters are more resistant to rupture. Histologically, bullous pemphigoid shows subepidermal blister formation.

3. Epidermolysis bullosa: Epidermolysis bullosa (EB) is a group of inherited disorders characterized by extreme skin fragility. It is caused by defects in the proteins responsible for anchoring the epidermis to the underlying dermis. EB can be classified into four major types: simplex, junctional, dystrophic, and Kindler syndrome. Each subtype has specific clinical and histological features.

4. Dermatitis herpetiformis: Dermatitis herpetiformis is a chronic autoimmune blistering disease associated with gluten sensitivity. It is characterized by intensely itchy, grouped vesicles and papules on the extensor surfaces. Histologically, it shows subepidermal blister formation with neutrophilic infiltrates.

5. Linear IgA bullous dermatosis: Linear IgA bullous dermatosis is a rare autoimmune blistering disorder characterized by the linear deposition of IgA along the basement membrane zone. It typically presents as grouped blisters or urticarial plaques. Histologically, it shows subepidermal blister formation with neutrophilic infiltrates and linear IgA deposits.

Diagnosing bullous diseases requires a combination of clinical, histological, and immunofluorescence examination. Treatment options vary depending on the specific condition and may include topical or systemic corticosteroids, immunosuppressants, or biologic agents. Additionally, patient education and support are crucial for managing these chronic conditions.

As students in dermatology, it is important to recognize the clinical features and histological findings associated with bullous diseases. Familiarity with these conditions allows for accurate diagnosis, appropriate management, and improved patient care.

Chapter 9: Special Techniques in Dermatopathology

Immunohistochemistry in Dermatopathology

Immunohistochemistry (IHC) is a powerful technique used in dermatopathology to identify specific proteins in skin tissue samples. It plays a crucial role in the diagnosis and classification of various dermatological conditions. This subchapter will introduce students to the fundamentals of immunohistochemistry in dermatopathology, its applications, and its significance in the field of dermatology.

In dermatopathology, IHC aids in the identification of specific antigens or markers within skin cells. By using specific antibodies that bind to these markers, dermatopathologists can visualize the presence, location, and distribution of these proteins. This information is invaluable in determining the type of skin lesion, differentiating between various skin disorders, and assessing disease severity.

IHC has a wide range of applications in dermatopathology. It can be used to diagnose and classify different types of skin cancers, such as melanoma, basal cell carcinoma, and squamous cell carcinoma. By identifying specific markers associated with these cancers, dermatopathologists can accurately differentiate between benign and malignant lesions. Additionally, IHC can help evaluate the prognosis and response to treatment in skin cancer patients.

Furthermore, IHC is instrumental in the diagnosis of autoimmune blistering diseases, such as pemphigus and bullous pemphigoid. By identifying autoantibodies and immune complexes in skin samples, dermatopathologists can confirm the presence of these diseases and guide appropriate treatment strategies.

In the field of dermatology, IHC is also essential for studying inflammatory skin conditions like psoriasis, lupus erythematosus, and dermatitis. By analyzing the expression of specific markers, dermatopathologists can gain insights into the underlying immunological processes driving these diseases. This knowledge is crucial for developing targeted therapies and improving patient outcomes.

Understanding immunohistochemistry is vital for students studying dermatopathology. By learning the principles and techniques of IHC, students can accurately interpret and analyze immunostained slides. They will acquire the skills needed to identify important markers and understand their significance in different dermatological conditions. Furthermore, students will develop a solid foundation for conducting their own research and contributing to advancements in the field of dermatopathology.

In conclusion, immunohistochemistry is a valuable tool in dermatopathology that aids in the diagnosis, classification, and understanding of various skin disorders. Students studying dermatology will greatly benefit from understanding the principles and applications of IHC. By incorporating this technique into their practice, they can enhance their diagnostic accuracy and contribute to the advancement of dermatopathology.

Molecular Pathology in Dermatopathology

In recent years, molecular pathology has emerged as a valuable tool in the field of dermatopathology. This subchapter aims to provide students in the field of dermatology with a comprehensive understanding of the role of molecular pathology in the diagnosis, prognosis, and treatment of dermatological conditions.

Molecular pathology involves the study of genetic and molecular abnormalities within cells and tissues. By analyzing the molecular changes that occur in dermatological diseases, dermatopathologists can gain crucial insights into the underlying mechanisms and develop targeted therapies.

One of the key applications of molecular pathology in dermatopathology is in the diagnosis of skin cancers. By identifying specific genetic mutations or alterations, dermatopathologists can accurately differentiate between benign and malignant lesions. For example, the detection of BRAF mutations is highly indicative of melanoma, allowing for early intervention and improved patient outcomes.

Furthermore, molecular pathology plays a vital role in predicting the prognosis of dermatological conditions. By examining genetic biomarkers, dermatopathologists can assess the likelihood of disease progression, metastasis, and patient survival. This information is invaluable in determining the most appropriate treatment plan and guiding patient management.

In addition to diagnosis and prognosis, molecular pathology also contributes to the development of targeted therapies in dermatology.

By identifying genetic mutations or aberrant signaling pathways, researchers can design drugs that specifically target these abnormalities. This personalized approach to treatment has revolutionized dermatology, leading to improved outcomes and reduced side effects for patients.

To fully grasp the potential of molecular pathology in dermatopathology, students must familiarize themselves with the techniques and methodologies used in this field. These include polymerase chain reaction (PCR), fluorescence in situ hybridization (FISH), and next-generation sequencing (NGS). By understanding these techniques, students can effectively interpret molecular pathology reports and contribute to the advancement of dermatological research.

In conclusion, molecular pathology has become an integral part of dermatopathology, offering valuable insights into diagnosis, prognosis, and treatment. Students in the field of dermatology must recognize the immense potential of molecular pathology and stay updated with the latest advancements in this rapidly evolving field. By embracing molecular pathology, future dermatopathologists can significantly enhance their ability to provide accurate diagnoses, prognoses, and personalized treatment options for their patients.

Electron Microscopy in Dermatopathology

In the field of dermatopathology, electron microscopy plays a crucial role in providing detailed insights into the ultrastructure of various skin diseases. This subchapter aims to introduce students to the principles and applications of electron microscopy in dermatology, enabling them to better understand the microscopic characteristics of skin disorders.

Electron microscopy involves the use of an electron microscope, which utilizes a beam of electrons instead of light to visualize specimens at a much higher resolution. This technology allows for the examination of cellular and tissue structures with incredible detail, providing a deeper understanding of the pathological changes occurring in the skin.

One of the primary applications of electron microscopy in dermatopathology is the evaluation of skin biopsies. By examining the ultrastructural features of skin cells and their components, electron microscopy can help identify various diseases such as bullous disorders, metabolic diseases, and connective tissue disorders. It can also aid in the diagnosis of viral, bacterial, and fungal infections affecting the skin.

Students will learn about the different techniques used in electron microscopy, including the preparation of skin samples for examination. This includes fixation, dehydration, embedding, and sectioning of tissue specimens. They will gain an understanding of the advantages and limitations of electron microscopy compared to other diagnostic techniques like light microscopy and immunohistochemistry.

Furthermore, the subchapter will delve into the interpretation of electron micrographs, acquainting students with the various cellular and subcellular structures encountered in dermatopathology. They will learn to identify characteristic features such as desmosomes, tonofilaments, melanosomes, and basement membrane abnormalities, which are essential in diagnosing specific skin conditions.

Case studies and clinical correlations will be provided to illustrate the practical application of electron microscopy in dermatopathology. Students will be exposed to real-world scenarios, allowing them to apply their knowledge and critical thinking skills in analyzing electron micrographs and formulating accurate diagnoses.

By the end of this subchapter, students will have a solid foundation in electron microscopy in dermatopathology. They will understand the benefits of electron microscopy in diagnosing skin diseases and be able to appreciate its complementary role in conjunction with other diagnostic modalities. This knowledge will equip them with valuable skills as they progress in their studies and careers in dermatology.

Chapter 10: Dermatopathology in Clinical Practice

Dermatopathology in Dermatology Clinics

As students interested in the field of dermatology, it is essential to understand the crucial role that dermatopathology plays in diagnosing and treating skin diseases. Dermatopathology refers to the study of skin disorders through the examination of skin tissue samples under a microscope. It combines the expertise of both dermatologists and pathologists to accurately diagnose and classify various skin conditions.

In dermatology clinics, dermatopathology serves as a vital tool for diagnosing skin diseases accurately. When a patient presents with a skin lesion or a rash, dermatologists often take a biopsy of the affected area. This tissue sample is then sent to a dermatopathology laboratory for further analysis. The dermatopathologist examines the sample and provides a detailed report to the dermatologist, aiding in the formulation of an accurate diagnosis.

The information obtained from dermatopathology is crucial in determining appropriate treatment plans. By examining the skin tissue at a microscopic level, dermatopathologists can identify specific cellular changes, inflammatory responses, and abnormal growth patterns that help differentiate between various skin diseases. This knowledge is invaluable in determining the most effective treatment options, including topical creams, oral medications, or surgical interventions.

Moreover, dermatopathology plays a significant role in monitoring the progression of skin diseases and evaluating the effectiveness of treatment. By conducting follow-up biopsies, dermatopathologists can assess changes in the skin tissue and evaluate if the prescribed treatment is yielding positive results. This information guides further adjustments in the treatment plan, ensuring optimal patient care.

For students interested in pursuing a career in dermatology, a solid understanding of dermatopathology is essential. It provides a comprehensive insight into the underlying pathophysiology of skin diseases, allowing for accurate diagnoses and appropriate treatment recommendations. By learning to interpret microscopic findings, students can enhance their diagnostic skills and develop a more holistic approach to patient care.

Furthermore, knowledge of dermatopathology enables students to effectively communicate with dermatopathologists and pathologists, fostering a collaborative approach in patient management. This interdisciplinary collaboration is crucial in providing patients with the best possible care, as the expertise of both dermatologists and dermatopathologists is combined to deliver an accurate diagnosis and an appropriate treatment plan.

In conclusion, dermatopathology is an integral part of dermatology clinics, aiding in the diagnosis and management of various skin diseases. Students aspiring to be dermatologists must familiarize themselves with the principles of dermatopathology to enhance their diagnostic acumen and provide optimal patient care. By understanding the microscopic changes that occur in skin tissue, students can contribute to the interdisciplinary approach required for successful dermatological practice.

Dermatopathology in Surgical Pathology

Dermatopathology is a specialized field within the realm of pathology that focuses on the study of skin diseases. It plays a crucial role in the diagnosis, treatment, and management of various dermatological conditions. In this subchapter, we will delve into the significance of dermatopathology within the broader field of surgical pathology, providing students with a comprehensive understanding of its importance.

Surgical pathology involves the examination of tissue samples obtained during surgical procedures to diagnose diseases and guide treatment decisions. Dermatopathologists specialize in the analysis of skin samples, including biopsies and excisions, to identify and classify skin disorders. Their expertise is pivotal in distinguishing between benign and malignant conditions, determining disease progression, and formulating appropriate treatment plans.

For students pursuing a career in dermatology, understanding dermatopathology is crucial. It allows them to interpret histopathological findings and correlate them with clinical presentations. By analyzing microscopic features of skin lesions, dermatopathologists can provide valuable insights into the underlying pathology, aiding dermatologists in making accurate diagnoses and recommending suitable therapies.

This subchapter will provide students with an overview of the techniques and methodologies employed in dermatopathology. It will explore the process of specimen collection, fixation, and processing, as well as the staining and microscopy techniques used to examine skin samples. Students will gain a comprehensive understanding of the various histopathological patterns observed in different skin diseases, such as inflammatory, neoplastic, and infectious conditions.

Moreover, this subchapter will cover key diagnostic challenges frequently encountered in dermatopathology. It will address the importance of clinicopathological correlation, emphasizing the significance of integrating clinical history, physical examination findings, and laboratory investigations with histopathological analysis. Students will learn to recognize common pitfalls and avoid misinterpretations that may lead to diagnostic errors.

Furthermore, this subchapter will shed light on the critical role of molecular pathology in dermatopathology. It will introduce students to the emerging field of molecular diagnostics, exploring the use of molecular techniques to identify genetic alterations associated with various skin diseases. Understanding these advancements will enable students to stay abreast of the latest developments in the field and appreciate their potential for improving diagnostic accuracy and personalized patient care.

In conclusion, dermatopathology is an integral component of surgical pathology, particularly in the field of dermatology. This subchapter aims to equip students with the necessary knowledge and skills to appreciate the importance of dermatopathology in diagnosing and managing skin diseases. By understanding the intricacies of histopathological analysis, students will be well-prepared to embark on a successful career in dermatology, ensuring optimal patient care and outcomes.

Dermatopathology in Research

In the field of dermatology, dermatopathology plays a crucial role in advancing our understanding of various skin diseases and disorders. This subchapter aims to provide students with a comprehensive overview of dermatopathology in research and its significance in the field of dermatology.

Dermatopathology refers to the study of skin diseases under a microscope, combining the disciplines of dermatology and pathology. Through this specialized branch of medicine, researchers are able to examine skin tissue samples and identify the underlying causes and characteristics of various skin conditions. By analyzing these samples, dermatopathologists can provide valuable insights into the diagnosis, prognosis, and treatment options for patients.

Research in dermatopathology encompasses a wide range of areas, including studying the histopathological features of skin diseases, investigating the molecular mechanisms involved in skin disorders, and exploring novel therapeutic interventions. By conducting research in dermatopathology, students can contribute to the development of new diagnostic tools, treatment strategies, and preventive measures for various dermatological conditions.

One of the key aspects of dermatopathology research is the correlation between clinical and histopathological findings. Students will learn how to integrate clinical information, such as patient history, physical examination, and laboratory tests, with the microscopic examination of skin specimens. This correlation is essential for accurate diagnosis and optimal patient care.

Furthermore, this subchapter will delve into the role of immunohistochemistry and molecular techniques in dermatopathology research. Students will gain an understanding of how these advanced techniques can be used to identify specific markers, determine the origin of tumors, and predict prognosis. The integration of these techniques with traditional histopathology provides a comprehensive approach to studying skin diseases and contributes to the development of personalized medicine.

Lastly, students will explore the ethical considerations and challenges faced in dermatopathology research. This subchapter will discuss the importance of obtaining informed consent from patients, maintaining privacy and confidentiality, and adhering to ethical guidelines in conducting research involving human subjects.

By studying dermatopathology in research, students will gain a deeper understanding of the complex nature of skin diseases and contribute to advancements in the field of dermatology. This subchapter aims to equip students with the knowledge and skills necessary to critically analyze and contribute to the growing body of dermatopathology research.

Chapter 11: Case Studies in Dermatopathology

Case Study 1: Inflammatory Skin Disorder

Introduction:
In the field of dermatology, the study of inflammatory skin disorders is crucial for understanding various skin conditions that can affect individuals of all ages. This chapter aims to provide students with a comprehensive case study focusing on a specific inflammatory skin disorder, shedding light on its clinical presentation, diagnostic methods, and treatment options.

Case   Presentation:
Our case study revolves around a 35-year-old female patient who presented with persistent redness, itching, and swelling on her face. The symptoms had gradually worsened over the past few months, negatively impacting her self-esteem and overall quality of life. Upon examination, the dermatologist noticed erythematous papules and pustules primarily affecting the central face, along with telangiectasias and occasional nodules.

Diagnostic   Workup:
To establish a definitive diagnosis, several diagnostic tools were employed. Firstly, a thorough medical history was obtained, focusing on the onset and progression of symptoms, any known triggers, and the patient's medical background. Dermatoscopy, a non-invasive technique, was used to examine the skin lesions more closely, revealing characteristic features like follicular plugs and central red spots. Additionally, a skin biopsy was performed, and the specimen was sent for histopathological examination.

Histopathological Findings:
The histopathological analysis revealed findings consistent with rosacea, an inflammatory skin disorder. Microscopic examination demonstrated dilated blood vessels near the surface of the skin, perifollicular lymphocytic infiltrate, and increased sebaceous gland activity. These findings confirmed the diagnosis of papulopustular rosacea, one of the subtypes of this disorder.

Treatment and Management:
Following the diagnosis, a multi-faceted treatment approach was initiated. The patient was advised to adopt a gentle skincare routine, avoiding harsh products and excessive sun exposure. Topical medications, such as metronidazole and azelaic acid, were prescribed to control the inflammatory response and reduce the appearance of papules and pustules. In addition, lifestyle modifications, including stress reduction techniques and dietary changes, were recommended to manage triggers and prevent flare-ups.

Conclusion:
This case study presents a comprehensive overview of the clinical presentation, diagnostic workup, and treatment options for inflammatory skin disorders, focusing on a specific case of rosacea. Understanding the intricacies of such conditions is vital for students pursuing dermatology, as it equips them with the knowledge necessary to accurately diagnose and effectively manage these disorders. By studying real-life cases like this, students can develop a deeper understanding of dermatopathology and provide optimal care to their future patients.

Case Study 2: Infectious Skin Condition

In the field of dermatology, infectious skin conditions are a common occurrence that requires careful diagnosis and treatment. Understanding these conditions is crucial for students studying dermatopathology, as they will encounter numerous cases throughout their careers. In this case study, we will explore an interesting infectious skin condition, highlighting its causes, symptoms, and treatment options.

Title: A Closer Look at Impetigo: A Common Contagious Skin Infection

Introduction:
Impetigo, a highly contagious bacterial skin infection, primarily affects children but can occur in individuals of all ages. This condition is caused by either Staphylococcus aureus or Streptococcus pyogenes bacteria. Understanding the clinical presentation, diagnostic methods, and treatment options for impetigo is essential for dermatology students.

Clinical   Presentation:
Impetigo typically begins with the appearance of small, red sores that rapidly transform into blisters, which eventually rupture and leave behind a yellowish-brown crust. These lesions are mostly found on the face, hands, and other exposed areas of the body. Itching and pain are common symptoms, often leading to scratching, which can further spread the infection.

Diagnosis:
To diagnose impetigo, a thorough physical examination is usually

sufficient. However, in certain cases, a laboratory analysis of a fluid sample obtained from the blister may be necessary to identify the causative bacteria. This helps determine the most effective treatment strategy.

Treatment:

The treatment of impetigo involves both topical and oral antibiotics. Mild cases can often be managed with topical antibiotic ointments, such as mupirocin, applied directly to the affected areas. However, more severe cases may require oral antibiotics, such as penicillin or erythromycin, to effectively eliminate the infection.

Prevention and Control:

Since impetigo is highly contagious, proper hygiene practices play a crucial role in its prevention. Regular handwashing, avoiding close contact with infected individuals, and keeping personal belongings clean can significantly reduce the risk of transmission. Additionally, prompt treatment and isolation of infected individuals can help prevent the spread of impetigo.

Conclusion:

Impetigo is a common infectious skin condition that primarily affects children. Dermatology students should familiarize themselves with its clinical presentation, diagnostic methods, and treatment options. By understanding the causes, symptoms, and appropriate management of impetigo, students will be better equipped to diagnose and treat similar infectious skin conditions throughout their careers.

Case Study 3: Neoplastic Skin Condition

In this chapter, we will delve into a fascinating case study that explores the intricate world of neoplastic skin conditions. Neoplastic skin conditions refer to abnormal growths or tumors that arise from the skin or its appendages. These conditions can present a significant challenge for dermatologists, making it crucial for students of dermatology to understand their clinical presentation, diagnostic approach, and management strategies.

Our case study revolves around a patient who presented with a suspicious skin lesion on their forearm. Upon examination, the lesion appeared as a well-defined, raised, and pigmented nodule. The dermatologist noted that it had irregular borders and variations in color, which raised concerns about its potentially malignant nature. To confirm the diagnosis, a skin biopsy was performed.

The histopathological examination of the biopsy revealed the presence of atypical melanocytes within the epidermis and dermis, forming nests and extending into the surrounding tissue. The presence of these abnormal cells confirmed the diagnosis of malignant melanoma, a type of skin cancer that arises from melanocytes.

Melanoma is a highly aggressive and potentially lethal form of skin cancer. It requires prompt and comprehensive management to achieve the best patient outcomes. The dermatologist discussed the case with a multidisciplinary team, including surgical oncologists and dermatopathologists, to develop an appropriate treatment plan.

Treatment options for melanoma depend on various factors, such as the tumor thickness, depth of invasion, and presence of metastasis. In this case, the dermatologist recommended surgical excision of the lesion, followed by sentinel lymph node biopsy to assess the spread of the cancer. The patient was also advised to undergo regular follow-ups and self-examinations to monitor for any recurrence or new lesions.

This case study highlights the importance of early detection and proper management of neoplastic skin conditions. As future dermatologists, it is crucial for students to develop a comprehensive understanding of the clinical and histopathological features of various skin tumors. By doing so, they will be better equipped to make accurate diagnoses and provide appropriate treatment plans to their patients.

In conclusion, this case study serves as a valuable learning experience for students of dermatology, shedding light on the intricate world of neoplastic skin conditions. By studying and understanding cases like this, students can enhance their diagnostic skills and develop effective management approaches for their future patients.

Case Study 4: Autoimmune and Connective Tissue Disorder

Case Study 4: Autoimmune and Connective Tissue Disorders

Introduction:
In the field of dermatology, autoimmune and connective tissue disorders present a unique set of challenges for both diagnosis and treatment. This case study aims to provide students with a comprehensive understanding of these disorders, their clinical presentations, and histopathological features.

1.   Systemic   Lupus   Erythematosus   (SLE): SLE is a chronic autoimmune disease that affects multiple organs, including the skin. Students will explore the clinical manifestations of SLE, such as the characteristic butterfly rash and systemic symptoms. Histopathological findings, including interface dermatitis and deposition of immunoglobulin and complement, will be discussed. Diagnostic criteria and treatment options will also be covered.

2.   Dermatomyositis   (DM): DM is a rare connective tissue disorder characterized by muscle weakness and skin manifestations. This case study will highlight the classical cutaneous findings, including Gottron's papules and heliotrope rash. Histopathological examination will focus on perifascicular atrophy and presence of inflammatory infiltrates. Students will learn about associated conditions, such as malignancies, and the importance of early recognition and treatment.

3.   Scleroderma: Scleroderma is a group of autoimmune disorders characterized by fibrosis and thickening of the skin. Students will explore the two main

subtypes: limited cutaneous systemic sclerosis and diffuse cutaneous systemic sclerosis. Clinical manifestations, including Raynaud's phenomenon and sclerodactyly, will be discussed. Histopathological features, such as collagen deposition and vascular changes, will be examined. Treatment options, including immunosuppressive agents and supportive care, will also be covered.

4.   Mixed Connective Tissue Disease (MCTD): MCTD is a rare autoimmune disorder that combines features of several connective tissue diseases. This case study will focus on the clinical and histopathological aspects of MCTD, including the presence of anti-U1 RNP antibodies. Students will learn about the challenges in diagnosing MCTD due to overlapping clinical features and the importance of multidisciplinary management.

Conclusion:

Understanding autoimmune and connective tissue disorders is crucial for students pursuing a career in dermatology. This case study has provided an overview of SLE, DM, scleroderma, and MCTD, including their clinical presentations and histopathological features. By familiarizing themselves with these disorders, students will be better equipped to diagnose and manage patients with autoimmune and connective tissue disorders in their future practice.

Chapter 12: Future Directions in Dermatopathology

Advances in Dermatopathological Techniques

Dermatopathology is a specialized field within dermatology that focuses on the study and diagnosis of skin diseases through the examination of skin biopsies. Over the years, significant advances have been made in dermatopathological techniques, revolutionizing the way skin diseases are diagnosed and treated. In this subchapter, we will explore some of these advancements and their implications for students in the field of dermatology.

One of the most noteworthy advances in dermatopathology is the introduction of immunohistochemistry (IHC) staining techniques. IHC allows dermatopathologists to detect specific proteins or antigens within skin tissue, aiding in the identification of different cell types and their characteristics. This technique has greatly enhanced the accuracy and specificity of diagnoses, enabling more targeted treatment plans for patients. Students should familiarize themselves with the various IHC markers commonly used in dermatopathology, as they play a crucial role in distinguishing between different skin disorders.

Another significant advancement is the use of molecular techniques in dermatopathology. Polymerase chain reaction (PCR) and fluorescence in situ hybridization (FISH) are two commonly employed molecular methods that allow for the detection of specific gene mutations or chromosomal abnormalities associated with certain skin diseases. These techniques have revolutionized the diagnosis and classification of many skin conditions, particularly those with a genetic basis. By understanding the principles and limitations of molecular techniques, students can effectively utilize these tools to provide accurate diagnoses and help guide treatment decisions.

Digital pathology is yet another breakthrough that has transformed the field of dermatopathology. With the advent of whole-slide imaging (WSI) scanners, glass slides containing skin biopsies can now be digitized and viewed on a computer screen. This technology has facilitated remote consultations, collaboration between pathologists, and the creation of comprehensive digital archives. Students should familiarize themselves with the technical aspects of WSI, as well as the potential benefits and challenges associated with its implementation in dermatopathology practice.

Lastly, the integration of artificial intelligence (AI) and machine learning algorithms has shown promising results in dermatopathology. These technologies can aid in the automated analysis of digitized slides, assisting pathologists in the interpretation and classification of skin diseases. Students should stay updated on the latest advancements in AI and machine learning, as they have the potential to enhance diagnostic accuracy, increase efficiency, and improve patient care.

In conclusion, dermatopathology has witnessed remarkable advancements in recent years. From immunohistochemistry and molecular techniques to digital pathology and AI, these innovations have revolutionized the field and transformed how skin diseases are diagnosed and managed. As students in the field of dermatology, understanding and embracing these advances will be essential in providing accurate diagnoses and delivering optimal patient care.

Emerging Trends in Dermatopathology Research

As students pursuing a career in dermatology, it is crucial to stay updated on the latest advancements and emerging trends in dermatopathology research. The field of dermatopathology is constantly evolving, and new discoveries are being made that have the potential to revolutionize the diagnosis and treatment of various skin conditions. In this subchapter, we will explore some of the most significant emerging trends in dermatopathology research.

One of the prominent trends in dermatopathology research is the use of molecular diagnostics. Advances in technology now allow for the identification of specific genetic mutations and alterations that play a crucial role in the development and progression of skin diseases. By analyzing these molecular markers, dermatopathologists can provide more accurate diagnoses and develop personalized treatment plans tailored to each patient's unique genetic makeup.

Another emerging trend is the integration of artificial intelligence (AI) and machine learning in dermatopathology. AI algorithms can analyze vast amounts of data, including histopathological images, to identify patterns and make predictions with high accuracy. This technology has the potential to assist dermatopathologists in diagnosing skin diseases more efficiently and improving patient outcomes.

Furthermore, there is a growing interest in studying the role of the skin microbiome in dermatopathology. The skin is home to a diverse community of microorganisms that interact with the host's immune system and play a significant role in maintaining skin health. Research in this area aims to understand how alterations in the skin microbiome contribute to the development of various skin disorders and how manipulating the microbiome can be used as a therapeutic approach.

In addition to these technological advancements, there is a renewed focus on dermatopathology research related to skin cancer. With the rising incidence of skin cancer worldwide, there is a need for improved diagnostic tools and targeted therapies. Researchers are exploring novel biomarkers, such as specific gene mutations or protein expressions, that can aid in the early detection and treatment of skin cancer.

Overall, these emerging trends in dermatopathology research hold immense potential for the future of dermatology. As students, it is vital to stay informed and actively engage in this evolving field. By embracing these advancements, we can contribute to improving patient care, enhancing diagnostic accuracy, and developing innovative treatment strategies for a wide range of dermatological conditions.

Role of Artificial Intelligence in Dermatopathology

Artificial Intelligence (AI) has made significant advancements in various fields, and dermatopathology is no exception. Dermatology students can greatly benefit from understanding the role of AI in their field. This subchapter aims to explore the potential of AI in dermatopathology and its impact on the field of dermatology.

Dermatopathology involves the study of skin disorders by integrating clinical information with microscopic examination of skin specimens. This process requires expertise and experience, as dermatologists need to accurately diagnose diseases based on histological findings. However, the interpretation of skin biopsies can be challenging and time-consuming, leading to potential errors or delays in diagnoses.

AI technology offers a promising solution to these challenges. By analyzing vast amounts of data, AI algorithms can assist dermatologists in diagnosing skin diseases more accurately and efficiently. Machine learning algorithms can be trained to recognize patterns and identify key features in microscopic images, allowing for enhanced diagnostic accuracy. This can help students in dermatology gain valuable insights and improve their diagnostic abilities.

Furthermore, AI can assist in the early detection of skin cancers, such as melanoma. With the ability to analyze images and recognize suspicious lesions, AI algorithms can aid in identifying potential malignancies at an early stage. This early detection can save lives and improve patient outcomes. Dermatology students can leverage AI technology to enhance their skills in identifying melanoma and other skin cancers, ultimately improving patient care.

In addition to diagnosis and early detection, AI can also play a role in treatment planning. By analyzing patient data, AI algorithms can provide personalized treatment recommendations based on the individual's medical history, genetic profile, and response to previous therapies. Students can learn how to integrate AI-generated treatment plans into their practice, ensuring optimal patient care and outcomes.

Despite the potential benefits, it is important for students to understand the limitations of AI in dermatopathology. AI algorithms rely on training data, and biases within these datasets can lead to inaccurate diagnoses. Therefore, it is crucial for dermatology students to critically evaluate and validate AI-generated results to ensure patient safety and ethical practice.

In conclusion, AI holds immense potential in dermatopathology. Students pursuing dermatology can harness the power of AI to improve their diagnostic abilities, aid in early detection of skin cancers, and optimize treatment planning. However, it is essential for students to understand the limitations and ethical considerations associated with AI technology. By embracing AI advancements, dermatology students can stay at the forefront of their field and provide enhanced care to their patients.

Chapter 13: Resources for Further Learning

Books and Textbooks in Dermatopathology

As students pursuing a career in dermatology, it is crucial to have a solid understanding of dermatopathology. This subchapter aims to provide you with an overview of essential books and textbooks that will serve as valuable resources throughout your journey in this field.

1. "Dermatopathology: A Volume in the Foundations in Diagnostic Pathology Series" by Dirk Elston, Tammie Ferringer, and Christine J. Ko: This comprehensive textbook offers a systematic approach to dermatopathology, covering both common and rare dermatologic conditions. It features high-quality images, detailed discussions on diagnostic criteria, and practical tips for accurate interpretation. This book is an excellent starting point for students looking to build a strong foundation in dermatopathology.

2. "Dermatopathology: Expert Consult - Online and Print" by Elston, Ferringer, Ko, and William D. James: Another highly recommended textbook, this resource provides a detailed understanding of dermatopathology through a combination of text, high-resolution images, and online access to additional materials. It covers a wide range of skin diseases, including inflammatory, infectious, and neoplastic conditions. The book also includes quizzes and self-assessment tools to reinforce your knowledge.

3. "Dermatopathology: Diagnosis by First Impression" by Christine J. Ko, Ronald J. Barr, and Ronald P. Rapini: This unique textbook focuses on the importance of developing diagnostic skills based on

initial impressions. It emphasizes pattern recognition and correlation with clinical findings, helping students become more efficient and accurate in their diagnoses. The book also provides a practical approach to reporting and communicating dermatopathology findings.

4. "Dermatopathology: High-Yield Pathology" by Arthur R. Rhodes: Designed specifically for medical students and residents, this concise textbook delivers essential information in a user-friendly format. It covers the most important topics in dermatopathology, including common inflammatory and neoplastic conditions, as well as infectious diseases. The book's high-yield format makes it an excellent resource for exam preparation and quick reference.

5. "Atlas of Dermatopathology: Practical Differential Diagnosis" by Klaus J. Busam: This visually stunning atlas features a vast collection of clinical and histopathological images, facilitating the recognition and differentiation of various dermatologic conditions. It covers a wide range of diseases and includes helpful annotations to guide students through the diagnostic process. The book's practical approach and extensive image library make it an indispensable resource for dermatology students.

In conclusion, a thorough understanding of dermatopathology is essential for students pursuing a career in dermatology. The recommended books and textbooks in this subchapter provide comprehensive coverage of the subject, offering valuable insights, diagnostic criteria, and practical tips. By utilizing these resources, students can enhance their knowledge and develop the necessary skills to excel in the field of dermatopathology.

Online Resources and Websites

In today's digital age, online resources and websites have become invaluable tools for students in various fields of study, including dermatology. The field of dermatopathology, in particular, relies heavily on these resources to supplement traditional learning methods and provide students with access to a wealth of information that is just a click away.

When it comes to dermatology, online resources and websites offer students a myriad of benefits. Firstly, they provide quick and easy access to a vast amount of knowledge. Students can access online textbooks, academic journals, and research papers, allowing them to stay updated with the latest advancements in the field. This instant access eliminates the need to spend hours searching through physical books or waiting for materials to be delivered.

Additionally, online resources and websites often offer interactive learning tools that can enhance the educational experience. Students can find virtual atlases, image galleries, and case studies, which provide visual representations of various dermatological conditions. These resources enable students to develop a better understanding of the subject matter and enhance their diagnostic skills.

Moreover, online resources and websites offer platforms for discussion and collaboration. Students can join online forums or participate in webinars where they can connect with fellow students, dermatologists, and experts in the field. This interaction allows for the exchange of ideas, the opportunity to ask questions, and the chance to gain insights from experienced professionals.

Some notable online resources and websites that students in dermatology can explore include DermNet NZ, a comprehensive online dermatology resource that provides information on various skin conditions, treatment options, and educational materials. Another valuable resource is the American Academy of Dermatology (AAD) website, which offers a plethora of educational tools, including e-learning modules, clinical guidelines, and research articles.

In conclusion, online resources and websites have revolutionized the way students learn and access information in the field of dermatopathology. With their easy accessibility, interactive learning tools, and platforms for collaboration, these resources are essential for students in dermatology. By utilizing these resources effectively, students can enhance their knowledge, improve their diagnostic skills, and stay up-to-date with the latest advancements in the field.

Dermatopathology Conferences and Workshops

As students pursuing a career in dermatology, it is crucial to stay updated with the latest advancements and research in the field. One of the best ways to achieve this is by attending dermatopathology conferences and workshops. These events provide a platform for students to learn from renowned experts, network with professionals, and gain valuable insights into the field of dermatopathology.

Dermatopathology conferences bring together experts from various subfields of dermatology to discuss and present their research findings. These conferences typically feature keynote lectures, panel discussions, and poster presentations. Attending these lectures allows students to expand their knowledge base, learn about cutting-edge research, and understand the practical application of various diagnostic techniques.

Workshops, on the other hand, offer students a hands-on learning experience. These interactive sessions provide an opportunity to practice and enhance their skills in dermatopathology. Workshops may include activities like slide reviews, case discussions, and microscopy training. Participating in these workshops not only improves diagnostic accuracy but also helps students develop critical thinking and problem-solving abilities.

Apart from the educational aspect, dermatopathology conferences and workshops also serve as a networking platform. Students can interact with professionals, researchers, and fellow students who share a common interest in dermatology. Networking at these events can lead to collaborations, mentorship opportunities, and exposure to potential job prospects. Furthermore, engaging with experts in the field allows students to gain insights into career paths, research opportunities, and advancements in dermatopathology.

To make the most of these events, it is essential to plan ahead. Research the conference or workshop agenda, identify sessions that align with your interests, and set specific learning goals. Prepare questions and actively participate in discussions to make the most out of your experience. Additionally, consider presenting your own research or case study at these events to gain visibility and receive valuable feedback.

In conclusion, attending dermatopathology conferences and workshops is an excellent way for students to stay updated with the latest advancements in the field of dermatology. These events provide a platform to learn from experts, enhance practical skills, and network with professionals. By actively participating in these conferences and workshops, students can broaden their knowledge, gain valuable insights, and pave the way for a successful career in dermatopathology.

Chapter 14: Conclusion and Final Thoughts

Recap of Key Concepts

In this subchapter, we will review the fundamental concepts and principles that you have learned so far in "The Complete Guide to Dermatopathology for Students." As aspiring dermatologists, it is crucial to have a solid understanding of these key concepts to excel in your studies and future practice.

First and foremost, dermatopathology is the specialized field that combines dermatology and pathology. It involves the study of skin diseases at a microscopic level, enabling practitioners to diagnose and treat various dermatological conditions accurately. By analyzing skin tissue samples, dermatopathologists can identify specific cellular changes, inflammation, and other pathological features that aid in disease diagnosis.

One of the primary concepts in dermatopathology is the classification of skin diseases. Dermatologists use a systematic approach to categorize various dermatological conditions based on their clinical presentation, histopathological features, and underlying etiology. Understanding the classification system is crucial for accurate diagnosis and appropriate management of patients.

Another essential concept is the interpretation of histopathological slides. Dermatopathology relies heavily on the analysis of skin tissue samples under a microscope. Therefore, it is crucial to develop skills in recognizing and interpreting cellular structures, inflammatory patterns, and other microscopic features. This expertise will enable you to differentiate between different skin diseases and provide accurate diagnoses.

Furthermore, a comprehensive understanding of the normal structure and function of the skin is essential. Familiarize yourself with the different layers of the skin, including the epidermis, dermis, and subcutaneous tissue. Learn about the various cell types present in the skin, such as keratinocytes, melanocytes, and fibroblasts, and their roles in maintaining skin health.

Lastly, it is essential to keep up-to-date with the latest advancements and research in dermatopathology. Stay informed about emerging technologies, novel diagnostic techniques, and evolving treatment options. By staying current, you will be better equipped to provide optimal care to your patients and contribute to the advancement of the field.

In conclusion, this subchapter has provided a concise recap of the key concepts in dermatopathology. By understanding the fundamentals of dermatopathology, including disease classification, histopathological interpretation, normal skin structure and function, and staying informed about the latest advancements in the field, you will be well-prepared to excel in your studies and future career as a dermatologist.

Importance of Dermatopathology for Students

Dermatopathology is a crucial field of study for students pursuing a career in dermatology. As students, it is essential to understand the significance of dermatopathology and how it plays a vital role in diagnosing and treating various skin disorders. This subchapter aims to highlight the importance of dermatopathology for students in the field of dermatology.

Firstly, dermatopathology provides students with a comprehensive understanding of the pathological processes that occur in the skin. By examining skin biopsies under a microscope, students can observe the cellular and tissue changes associated with different skin conditions. This knowledge is crucial for accurate diagnosis and effective treatment planning.

Additionally, dermatopathology helps students develop essential skills in pattern recognition. By studying various dermatopathological slides, students can identify characteristic patterns and differentiate between various skin diseases. This skill is invaluable in clinical practice, where accurate diagnosis is vital for providing appropriate patient care.

Furthermore, dermatopathology equips students with the ability to communicate effectively with pathologists. Collaborating with pathologists is essential for obtaining accurate and timely diagnoses. By understanding the language and terminology of dermatopathology, students can effectively communicate their clinical findings and collaborate with pathologists to reach an accurate diagnosis.

Moreover, dermatopathology enhances students' critical thinking abilities. By analyzing complex histopathological slides, students learn to interpret and integrate clinical and histopathological findings, ultimately leading to accurate diagnoses. This skill is fundamental in dermatology, where diseases often present with overlapping clinical features.

Additionally, dermatopathology helps students stay updated with the latest advancements in the field. As the field of dermatology continues to evolve, new diagnostic techniques and treatments emerge. By studying dermatopathology, students can stay abreast of these advancements and integrate them into their clinical practice, providing the best possible care for their patients.

In conclusion, dermatopathology plays a crucial role in the education and training of students in the field of dermatology. It provides students with a comprehensive understanding of the pathological processes occurring in the skin, enhances their pattern recognition skills, improves critical thinking abilities, and keeps them updated with the latest advancements. By embracing dermatopathology, students can become competent dermatologists capable of accurately diagnosing and effectively treating various skin disorders.

Continuing Education in Dermatopathology for Students

In the ever-evolving field of dermatology, it is crucial for students to stay updated with the latest advancements and techniques in dermatopathology. Continuing education plays a vital role in ensuring that students are equipped with the necessary knowledge and skills to excel in this specialized area of dermatology. This subchapter will provide a comprehensive guide to help students understand the importance of continuing education in dermatopathology and the various resources available to them.

Continuing education serves as a bridge between academic learning and real-world practice. It allows students to expand their knowledge beyond the classroom and gain practical insights into the field of dermatopathology. By participating in continuing education programs, students can develop a deeper understanding of skin diseases, their histopathological features, and the diagnostic methods employed in dermatopathology.

One of the key benefits of continuing education in dermatopathology is the opportunity to learn from experienced professionals and experts in the field. Seminars, workshops, and conferences provide a platform for students to interact with renowned dermatopathologists, ask questions, and gain valuable insights into the challenges and advancements in this specialized area of dermatology.

Additionally, continuing education resources such as online courses, webinars, and self-study modules offer students the flexibility to learn at their own pace and convenience. These resources often include case studies, interactive quizzes, and virtual microscopy sessions, allowing students to enhance their diagnostic skills and improve their accuracy in identifying skin diseases.

Furthermore, staying updated with the latest research and developments in dermatopathology is essential for students to provide optimal patient care. Continuing education enables students to learn about emerging diagnostic techniques, novel treatment modalities, and advancements in molecular pathology. This knowledge empowers students to make informed decisions and deliver the highest standard of care to their patients.

In conclusion, continuing education plays a crucial role in the education and professional development of students in dermatopathology. By actively engaging in continuing education programs, students can enhance their diagnostic skills, stay updated with the latest advancements, and provide optimal care to patients. Whether through conferences, workshops, or online resources, students have a wide range of options to choose from to continue their education in dermatopathology. Embracing lifelong learning in this specialized field is essential to excel as a dermatopathologist and make a significant impact in the field of dermatology.